CHEST PAIN & HEART ATTACK

A Doctor's Guide to Recognizing Warning Signs, Acting Early & Protecting Your Life

---

Dr Prabhat Das

MD, PhD, FACP

Better Health with Dr Das Series

Hardcover ISBN: 978-1-971672-64-9

Paperback ISBN: 978-1-971672-63-2

eBook ISBN: 978-1-971672-62-5

Printed in the United States of America

Disclaimer

This book is intended solely for educational and informational purposes. It is not meant to replace personal medical advice, diagnosis, or treatment.

Although I am a licensed physician, reading this book does not establish a doctor-patient relationship. Each individual's health condition, medical history, and risk factors are unique. Any medical decision should be made in partnership with your own healthcare professional who understands your specific situation.

Medical science is continually advancing. New research and updated guidelines may lead to changes in recommendations over time.

TABLE OF CONTENTS:

About the Author

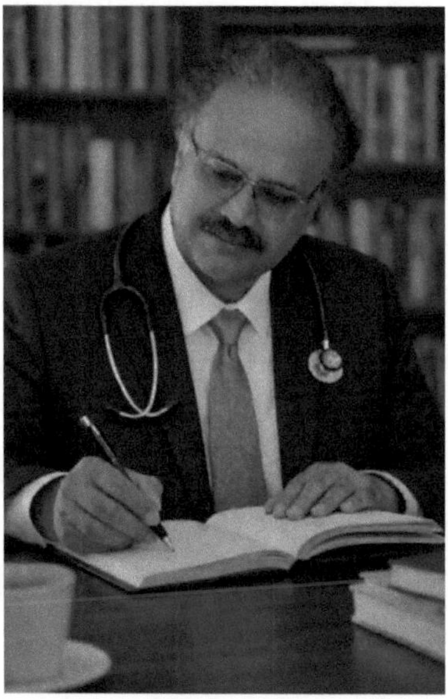

I am Dr Prabhat Das, MD, PhD, FACP. My journey in medicine began in India and, over the past thirty-five years, has continued in the United States, where I have had the privilege of caring for patients across a wide range of medical settings. I am trained in Internal Medicine, Pulmonary Diseases, and Critical Care. For me, medicine has never been just a profession. It has been a lifelong commitment shaped by learning, service, and a deep respect for the trust patients place in their physician.

Over the years, I have had the honor of caring for patients in many different situations. I have seen individuals in my office for routine concerns, treated urgent conditions in busy emergency rooms, managed serious illnesses in the hospital, and cared for critically ill patients in intensive care units. Each setting has taught me something valuable. Each patient has added to my understanding of what it truly means to care for another human being.

But one lesson has stood above all others. Medicine is not only about tests, diagnoses, or treatments. It is about people. It is about listening carefully, understanding fears that are often left unspoken, and guiding patients through uncertainty with clarity and compassion. Again and again, I have seen that what people want most is simple, trustworthy information. They want to understand what is happening in their bodies. They want to feel confident about the decisions they are making for their health and for their families.

These experiences have deeply shaped how I think about health, illness, prevention, and the human side of healing.

That is the reason behind the '**Better Health with Dr Das Series**'. Through these books, I hope to reach individuals I may never meet in person but who are searching for clear and reliable guidance. In today's world, health information is everywhere, yet much of it is confusing, overwhelming, and sometimes misleading. My goal is to cut through that noise and present important medical topics in a way that is simple, practical, and reassuring.

Every page of this series is guided by two foundations: reliable scientific knowledge and decades of real-world clinical experience. I want you, the reader, to feel informed, confident, and empowered. Not overwhelmed. Not confused. But clear about what you can do, step by step, to improve your health.

If even one reader feels less anxious, more informed, or better prepared to take control of their health after reading these books, then this work has served its purpose.

Helping people live healthier, longer, more confident and better-informed lives remains one of the greatest privileges of my life.

CHAPTER 1: Chest Pain After 40 — Why This Symptom Deserves Respect

Chest Pain Is Not an Ordinary Symptom

Chest pain is different.

A person may live with back pain for weeks, ignore a headache for days, or tolerate joint pain for months. But the moment discomfort appears in the chest, something changes inside us.

A quiet thought appears:

“Could this be my heart?”

That instinct is not wrong.

The heart works continuously, silently, without asking for attention. When it sends a signal, even a subtle one, it deserves to be taken seriously.

But here is where clarity matters.

Not every chest pain is a heart attack.
At the same time, some chest pain can be life-threatening.

The goal is not fear.
The goal is understanding and timely action.

CHAPTER 1

TYPES OF CHEST PAIN

HEART vs NON-HEART

Chest pain can have many causes.
It is important to understand the difference.

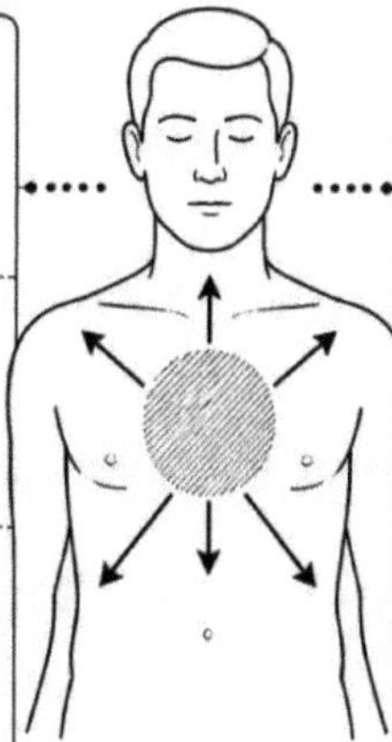

HEART-RELATED PAIN (POTENTIALLY SERIOUS)

PRESSURE / HEAVINESS
Feels like a weight or tight band on the chest.

RADIATES
May spread to arm, shoulder, neck, jaw or back.

ASSOCIATED SYMPTOMS
Sweating, shortness of breath, nausea, lightheadedness.

TRIGGERED BY EXEPTION / STRESS
Often brought on by activity or emotional stress and relieved by rest.

DURATION
Usually lasts more than a few minutes if untreated.

NON-HEART PAIN (USUALLY LESS SERIOUS)

SHARP / STABBING
Feels like a pin prick or knife-like pain.

LOCALIZED
Pain is in a small area. Does not spread.

FEW ASSOCIATED SYMPTOMS
Usually no sweating, breathlessness or nausea.

NOT RELATED TO EXERTION
Can occur at rest. May change with body movement, deep breath or touch.

DURATION
Often short-lived and comes and goes.

COMMON NON-HEART CAUSES

- Acidity / Acid reflux
- Muscle strain
- Rib or chest wall pain
- Lung problems
- Panic or anxiety
- Shingles

TAKEAWAY:
Not all chest pain is from the heart, but new, unusual or persistent pain should always be evaluated.

Why Chest Pain Is Often Misunderstood

One of the biggest challenges with chest pain is that it does not always behave the way people expect.

Many people imagine heart pain as sudden, severe, and unmistakable.

In reality, it is often described as:

- Pressure
- Heaviness
- Tightness
- A vague, uncomfortable feeling

Sometimes it is not even clearly felt in the chest. It may appear in:

- The arm
- The jaw
- The neck
- The back
- The upper abdomen

At times, the main symptoms may be:

- Shortness of breath
- Sweating
- Nausea
- Unusual fatigue

This variation creates confusion.

At the same time, common conditions such as acidity, muscle strain, or anxiety can produce similar symptoms.

That overlap is where mistakes happen.

Why Age 40 and Beyond Changes the Picture

After the age of 40, the risk of coronary artery disease increases steadily.

This risk becomes higher if a person has:

- High blood pressure
- Diabetes
- High cholesterol
- A history of smoking
- Excess body weight
- A family history of heart disease

This does not mean every chest discomfort is serious.

But it does mean something very important:

New, unusual, or unexplained chest symptoms should never be ignored.

In my practice, I often hear patients say:

"I thought it was just gas."

Sometimes they are right.

But sometimes, they are not.

And that difference can be life-changing.

The Hidden Danger of Waiting

A heart attack does not cause damage all at once.

It develops over time when blood flow to the heart is reduced or blocked.

The longer the delay:

- The more heart muscle is injured
- The more permanent the damage
- The greater the risk of complications

That is why we say:

Time is muscle.

This is not just a medical phrase. It is a real, practical truth.

Early action can preserve heart function.
Delay can change the course of a life.

A Real-Life Situation That Explains Everything

Let me share a situation I have seen many times.

A man in his late 50s feels a burning sensation in his chest after dinner. He assumes it is acidity. He takes medication. The discomfort improves slightly, but does not completely go away.

He goes to bed.

The next morning, he feels tired. While walking, he notices a mild heaviness in the chest. He ignores it and continues his routine.

By afternoon, the discomfort worsens. Now there is sweating and shortness of breath.

He finally seeks help.

Tests show a heart attack.

Now imagine a different decision.

The same patient takes the first symptom seriously and seeks medical care early. The artery is opened sooner. Less damage occurs. Recovery is smoother.

The difference is not luck.

The difference is timing.

Doctor's Pearl

Any new, unexplained, or changing chest discomfort should be treated seriously, especially after the age of 40 or in the presence of risk factors.

Common Mistakes to Avoid

- Assuming chest pain is always acidity
- Waiting for severe pain before acting
- Ignoring pressure or heaviness
- Trying home remedies first
- Feeling reassured because symptoms improve temporarily
- Underestimating symptoms in women or patients with diabetes

---

Red Flag Warnings

Seek immediate medical attention if chest discomfort is associated with:

- Pressure, tightness, or heaviness in the chest
- Pain spreading to the arm, jaw, neck, back, or upper abdomen
- Shortness of breath
- Sweating or cold, clammy skin
- Nausea or vomiting
- Dizziness or fainting
- Sudden, unexplained fatigue

Key Points

- Chest pain is a symptom, not a diagnosis
- It can arise from multiple causes, including the heart
- Heart-related discomfort is often not sharp pain
- After age 40, new symptoms deserve attention
- Early action can save heart muscle and life

Chapter Summary

Chest pain is one of the most important warning signals in medicine. While not every chest discomfort indicates a heart problem, it should never be ignored when it is new, unusual, or persistent. Heart-related symptoms often appear as pressure, heaviness, or breathlessness rather than sharp pain. Because these symptoms overlap with less serious conditions, self-diagnosis can be risky. The safest approach is awareness, early recognition, and timely medical evaluation.

Action Plan

- Pay attention to any new or unusual chest discomfort
- Do not assume it is acidity or stress
- Learn the warning signs of heart-related symptoms
- Call 911 if symptoms suggest a possible emergency
- Know your personal risk factors

- Seek medical advice for recurring or exertional symptoms

Bridge to the Next Chapter

You now understand why chest pain deserves respect.

The next question is even more important:

When should chest pain make you call 911 immediately?

In the next chapter, we will focus on the warning signs that should never be ignored.

CHAPTER 2: When Chest Pain Means Call 911 — Recognizing a True Emergency

One Decision That Can Change Everything

When chest discomfort begins, most people hesitate.

They wait.
They observe.
They hope it will go away.

This hesitation is human. But in heart disease, it can be dangerous.

The most important decision you will make is simple:

Do you act immediately, or do you wait?

I have seen both paths.

One patient calls 911 within minutes. Treatment begins early. Recovery is smooth.

Another waits, hoping the discomfort will pass. Hours go by. By the time help arrives, the damage is much greater.

The difference is often not the severity of the disease.

The difference is the timing of the decision.

What a Heart Emergency Really Feels Like

A heart attack does not always begin dramatically.

Many patients describe it in simple words:

- "It felt like pressure."
- "It was a heaviness."
- "Something just did not feel right."

The most common symptom is:

- Pressure, tightness, heaviness, or squeezing in the center of the chest

This discomfort may:

- Last several minutes or longer
- Come and go
- Gradually increase in intensity

It may spread to:

- One or both arms
- Neck or jaw
- Back or shoulders
- Upper abdomen

Symptoms That Should Never Be Ignored

Chest discomfort alone is important. But when it occurs with other symptoms, the concern increases.

Watch for:

- Shortness of breath
- Sweating
- Nausea or vomiting
- Lightheadedness or dizziness
- Sudden unusual fatigue
- A feeling of anxiety or uneasiness

In some people, especially women, older adults, and patients with diabetes, these symptoms may occur **without clear chest pain**.

This is where many heart attacks are missed.

Do Not Be Misled by Mild Symptoms

One of the most dangerous assumptions is:

"If it was serious, it would be severe."

This is not always true.

Many heart attacks begin with mild symptoms. Patients continue their routine, thinking it is nothing serious.

But inside the body, damage may already be occurring.

Mild symptoms do not mean a mild problem.

When Symptoms Come and Go

Another common situation is when symptoms improve temporarily.

Patients feel reassured and delay seeking help.

But heart-related discomfort can:

- Come and go
- Change in intensity
- Return later with greater severity

This pattern may represent unstable angina or an evolving heart attack.

Temporary relief should not delay action.

Why Calling 911 Is Critical

If you suspect a heart emergency, do not drive yourself.

This is very important.

While driving:

- Symptoms may worsen suddenly
- You may become dizzy or lose consciousness
- Treatment is delayed

Emergency medical services provide:

- Immediate monitoring
- Early treatment
- Faster access to hospital care

This can make a life-saving difference.

What To Do Immediately

If you or someone around you has symptoms suggestive of a heart attack:

- Call 911 immediately
- Stop all activity and sit or lie down
- Stay calm and avoid exertion
- If previously advised, chew an aspirin unless contraindicated
- Stay with someone until help arrives

Do not wait to see if symptoms improve.

A Real-Life Comparison

I remember a patient who told me:

"Doctor, I almost did not call. The pain was not that bad."

But he did call.

He reached the hospital early. Treatment was given quickly. His heart function remained strong.

Another patient delayed because the discomfort was mild.

By the time he arrived, significant heart damage had already occurred.

Once again, the difference was not luck.

The difference was action.

Doctor's Pearl

If you are unsure whether your symptoms are serious, treat them as serious until proven otherwise.

Common Mistakes to Avoid

- Waiting for symptoms to become severe
- Assuming it is acidity or gas
- Trying home remedies first
- Ignoring associated symptoms

- Driving yourself instead of calling emergency services
- Feeling reassured because symptoms improve temporarily

Red Flag Warnings

Call 911 immediately if you experience:

- Chest pressure, tightness, or heaviness lasting more than a few minutes
- Pain spreading to the arm, jaw, neck, back, or upper abdomen
- Shortness of breath
- Sweating, nausea, or dizziness
- Sudden unusual fatigue
- Any combination of these symptoms

Key Points

- Heart emergencies are not always dramatic
- Symptoms may be mild, intermittent, or unusual
- Delay increases heart damage
- Early action saves heart muscle and life

CHAPTER 2

WHEN TO CALL 911

EMERGENCY DECISION GUIDE

Chest **pain** can be a warning sign of a heart attack.
Use this guide to decide what to do.

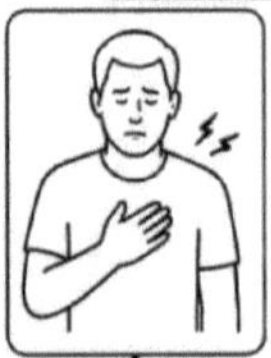

1 RECOGNIZE THE SYMPTOMS

- Chest pressure, tightness, or heaviness
- Pain spreading to arm, jaw, neck, back or upper abdomen
- Shortness of breath
- Sweating, nausea or dizziness

If you have any of these symptoms, go to **Step 2.**

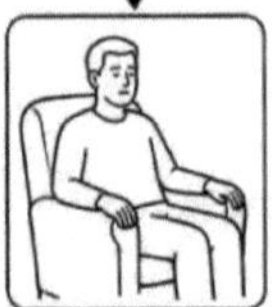

2 STOP AND REST

- Stop all activity immediately
- Sit or lie down
- Stay calm

If symptoms go away completely and do not return, monitor and consult your doctor.

If symptoms persist or worsen

3 CALL 911 IMMEDIATELY

- Do not wait to see if it improves
- Do not drive yourself
- Emergency medical care saves lives

EMS can start treatment right away and get you to the hospital safely.

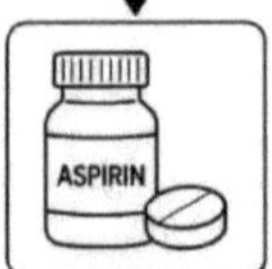

4 TAKE ASPIRIN (IF ADVISED)

- Chew one 325 mg aspirin if your doctor has advised it
- Do not take if allergic to aspirin or if advised not to take

Aspirin helps prevent clots and can reduce heart damage.

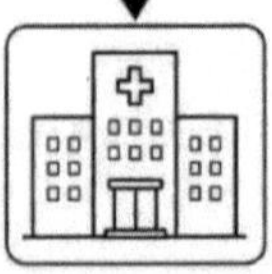

5 WAIT SAFELY FOR HELP

- Stay with someone if possible
- Monitor your symptoms
- Be ready to tell the paramedics your symptoms and history

Early treatment greatly improves outcomes.

WHAT NOT TO DO

- Do not ignore the pain
- Do not take home remedies first
- Do not wait for someone else to decide
- Do not delay calling 911

TAKEAWAY

When in doubt, treat chest pain as a heart emergency.
Act fast. Save life.

Chapter Summary

Recognizing a heart emergency is one of the most important life-saving skills. Chest discomfort, especially when associated with breathlessness, sweating, or radiation of pain, should never be ignored. Symptoms may be subtle or atypical, particularly in women, older adults, and patients with diabetes. Acting quickly and calling 911 can significantly reduce heart damage and improve survival.

Action Plan

- Learn and remember the warning signs
- Take any suspicious chest discomfort seriously
- Call 911 without delay when symptoms suggest an emergency
- Avoid self-treatment and waiting
- Educate your family about these warning signs

Bridge to the Next Chapter

You now know when chest pain becomes an emergency.

The next step is to understand what doctors mean when they use terms like coronary artery disease, angina, and heart attack.

In the next chapter, we will explain these clearly so that you can understand your condition with confidence.

CHAPTER 3: Coronary Artery Disease, Angina, and Heart Attack — Understanding the Connection Clearly

Why These Terms Create Confusion

In my daily practice, I often see more confusion than fear.

Patients hear different terms:

- Coronary artery disease
- Blocked arteries
- Angina
- Heart attack

Some think they all mean the same thing.
Others think they are completely different.

Both assumptions are incorrect.

Once you understand how these terms are connected, something important happens.

Fear is replaced by clarity.

You begin to see heart disease not as a sudden event, but as a process that develops over time.

CHAPTER 3

THE HEART DISEASE CONTINUUM

From Coronary Artery Disease to Heart Attack

Heart disease develops over many years.
Understanding this progression helps in early detection and prevention.

❶ CORONARY ARTERY DISEASE (CAD) → **❷ ANGINA** → **❸ HEART ATTACK**

❶ CORONARY ARTERY DISEASE (CAD)
The Beginning

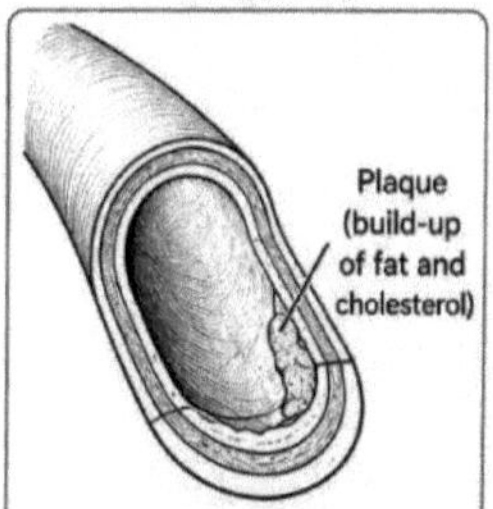

Plaque starts to build up inside the artery wall.
The artery is still open and blood flows normally.

❷ ANGINA
Reduced Blood Flow

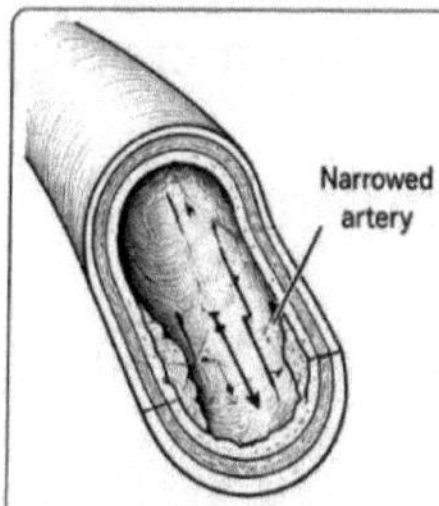

Plaque increases and narrows the artery.
During stress or activity, heart muscle may not get enough blood, causing chest pain (angina).

❸ HEART ATTACK
Complete Blockage

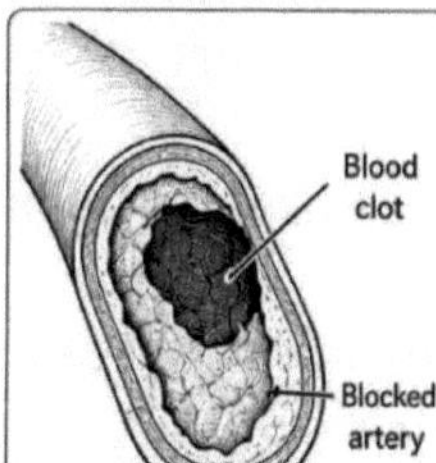

Plaque can rupture and a blood clot can form.
This can completely block the artery and cause a heart attack.

KEY POINTS

- The process starts years before any symptoms appear.
- Symptoms (like chest pain) usually start when the artery is significantly narrowed.
- A heart attack occurs when the artery suddenly becomes completely blocked.

TAKEAWAY
Heart attack does not happen suddenly without warning.
Early prevention and treatment can stop the progression and save your life.

HOW TO STOP THE PROGRESSION

- Quit Smoking
- Control Blood Pressure
- Control Diabetes
- Maintain Healthy Weight
- Eat Heart Healthy Diet
- Stay Active
- Regular Check-ups

Small steps today can prevent a major event tomorrow.

One Disease, Different Stages

Let me simplify this clearly.

Think of heart disease as a progression:

- Coronary artery disease → the underlying problem
- Angina → the warning signal
- Heart attack → the emergency event

These are not separate conditions.

They are different stages of the same disease process.

Coronary Artery Disease — The Silent Beginning

Coronary artery disease begins quietly.

The coronary arteries supply blood to the heart muscle. Over time, these arteries develop narrowing due to buildup of cholesterol, fatty material, and inflammatory cells.

This process is called atherosclerosis.

At this stage:

- You may feel completely normal
- There may be no symptoms

This is why coronary artery disease is often called a silent disease.

But silence does not mean safety.

The process is slowly progressing in the background.

Angina – The Heart's Early Warning

Angina is not a disease. It is a symptom.

It occurs when the heart muscle does not receive enough blood, especially during increased demand.

Patients usually describe it as:

- Pressure
- Heaviness
- Tightness
- A squeezing sensation

It typically occurs:

- During physical activity
- During emotional stress
- After heavy meals

And it usually improves with rest.

This pattern is very important.

It tells us that blood flow is reduced but not completely blocked.

Stable Angina and Unstable Angina — A Critical Difference

Understanding this difference can prevent serious outcomes.

Stable Angina

- Occurs with exertion
- Improves with rest
- Follows a predictable pattern

Many patients begin to ignore it because it is predictable.

That is a mistake.

It indicates significant narrowing in the arteries.

Unstable Angina

- Occurs at rest or with minimal activity
- Becomes more frequent
- Lasts longer
- Does not improve easily

This is dangerous.

It often means that a plaque has become unstable and may rupture.

A heart attack may follow.

Heart Attack — When Blood Flow Stops

A heart attack occurs when blood flow to a part of the heart is suddenly blocked.

This usually happens when:

- A plaque ruptures
- A blood clot forms rapidly

As a result:

- Oxygen supply to the heart muscle stops
- Damage begins within minutes
- If untreated, part of the heart muscle dies

This is a medical emergency.

How These Conditions Are Connected

Let us look at the sequence:

- Plaque builds up silently over years
- Blood flow becomes limited → angina
- Sudden blockage occurs → heart attack

Not every patient follows this exact sequence, but this is the most common pathway.

A Simple Everyday Example

Imagine a water pipe.

- Over time, deposits build up inside
- The pipe becomes narrower
- Water flow reduces when demand increases

This is like angina.

Now imagine a sudden blockage in the pipe.

- Water flow stops completely

This is like a heart attack.

The problem did not begin suddenly. It developed slowly.

Why This Understanding Matters

When you understand this process, you gain control.

You can:

- Recognize early warning signs
- Seek timely evaluation
- Prevent progression to a heart attack

You move from reacting to emergencies to preventing them.

Doctor's Pearl

Angina is not just discomfort. It is your heart asking for attention.

Common Mistakes to Avoid

- Ignoring angina because it improves with rest
- Assuming mild symptoms are not serious
- Confusing all chest pain with a heart attack
- Delaying evaluation of recurring symptoms

Red Flag Warnings

Seek urgent medical attention if:

- Chest discomfort occurs at rest
- Symptoms are increasing in frequency
- Pain lasts longer than usual

- Relief is incomplete
- Symptoms are associated with breathlessness or sweating

Key Points

- Coronary artery disease is the underlying problem
- Angina is a warning sign
- A heart attack occurs when blood flow is blocked
- These are stages of the same disease

Chapter Summary

Coronary artery disease develops silently over time due to narrowing of the coronary arteries. Angina appears when the heart muscle does not receive enough blood during increased demand. A heart attack occurs when a blockage suddenly becomes complete, leading to damage of the heart muscle. Understanding this progression helps in early recognition and timely prevention of serious outcomes.

Action Plan

- Learn to recognize angina symptoms
- Do not ignore recurring chest discomfort
- Seek medical evaluation early
- Understand your personal risk factors

- Act promptly when symptoms change

Bridge to the Next Chapter

Now that you understand what these conditions mean, the next question is:

Why do these blockages form in the first place?

In the next chapter, we will go inside the arteries and understand how plaque develops and what triggers a heart attack.

CHAPTER 4: Inside the Coronary Arteries — How Blockages Form and Why They Suddenly Become Dangerous

The Problem Begins Long Before Symptoms

One of the most important truths in heart disease is this:

The disease does not begin when chest pain starts.

It begins silently, often years or even decades earlier.

Patients often say, "This happened suddenly."

But in reality, the process has been developing quietly inside the arteries for a long time.

Understanding this process gives you something powerful:

The opportunity to prevent it.

What a Healthy Artery Looks Like

In a healthy state, the coronary arteries are:

- Smooth
- Flexible
- Wide enough for normal blood flow

Blood moves easily, supplying oxygen to the heart muscle.

The inner lining of the artery plays an important role. It helps regulate blood flow and keeps the vessel functioning normally.

When this lining is healthy, everything works smoothly.

The First Injury — Where It Starts

The process of heart disease usually begins with subtle injury to the inner lining of the artery.

Common causes include:

- High blood pressure
- High cholesterol
- Diabetes
- Smoking
- Chronic inflammation

Once this lining is damaged:

- Cholesterol enters the artery wall

- Inflammatory cells accumulate
- The body attempts repair, but the process is imperfect

This marks the beginning of plaque formation.

Plaque Formation — A Slow Process

Plaque is not just fat.

It is a mixture of:

- Cholesterol
- Fatty substances
- Inflammatory cells
- Calcium

Over time, plaque builds up inside the artery wall.

As it grows:

- The artery becomes narrower
- Blood flow becomes restricted
- The vessel becomes less flexible

At this stage, many people still have no symptoms.

Why This Is Not Just About Cholesterol

Many people believe heart disease is only about high cholesterol.

That is not entirely true.

Atherosclerosis is also an inflammatory process.

This means:

- The body's response to injury plays a key role
- Conditions like diabetes and smoking accelerate damage
- Even moderate cholesterol levels can become harmful in the presence of inflammation

This is why multiple risk factors together increase risk significantly.

Stable Plaque and Unstable Plaque

Not all plaques behave the same way.

Stable Plaque

- Develops slowly
- Has a thicker outer layer
- Less likely to rupture

- Often causes predictable symptoms such as stable angina

Unstable Plaque

- Has a thinner outer layer
- More prone to rupture
- May not cause severe narrowing
- Can trigger a sudden heart attack

This distinction is extremely important.

Plaque Rupture — The Critical Moment

Most heart attacks begin with plaque rupture.

When a fragile plaque breaks:

- Its contents are exposed to the bloodstream
- The body reacts as if there is an injury
- A blood clot forms rapidly

This clot can:

- Partially block the artery
- Completely block the artery

A complete blockage leads to a heart attack.

Why Even Small Blockages Can Be Dangerous

Patients often feel reassured when told they have "mild blockage."

But an important point must be understood:

Even smaller plaques can rupture and cause a heart attack.

Large plaques may cause gradual symptoms.

Smaller unstable plaques may cause sudden events.

Why Symptoms Often Appear Late

The body adapts over time.

As arteries narrow:

- Blood flow at rest may still be adequate
- Alternative pathways may develop

This is why:

- Many patients have no symptoms for years
- Symptoms appear only when demand increases

This delay can create a false sense of safety.

A Simple Example

Think of a highway.

- Over time, lanes become narrower
- Traffic still moves during light hours

During peak time:

- Traffic slows down

This is like angina.

Now imagine a sudden blockage.

- Traffic stops completely

This is like a heart attack.

The problem developed gradually, even though the event appears sudden.

Doctor's Pearl

Heart attacks are often caused by unstable plaques, not necessarily the largest blockages.

Common Mistakes to Avoid

- Thinking only severe blockages are dangerous
- Assuming no symptoms means no disease
- Ignoring risk factors
- Delaying preventive care

Red Flag Warnings

Be alert if:

- Chest discomfort becomes more frequent
- Symptoms occur with less activity
- Pain begins to occur at rest
- Relief becomes incomplete

These changes may signal an unstable condition.

Key Points

- Coronary artery disease develops slowly over time
- Plaque buildup narrows arteries
- Plaque rupture can cause sudden blockage
- Even small plaques can be dangerous

Chapter Summary

Atherosclerosis is a gradual process in which plaque builds up inside the coronary arteries. It begins with injury to the inner lining of the artery and progresses through accumulation of cholesterol and inflammatory material. Stable plaques may cause predictable symptoms, while unstable plaques can rupture suddenly, leading to clot formation and blockage of blood flow. This is the event that triggers a heart attack. Understanding this process highlights the importance of prevention and early intervention.

Action Plan

- Control blood pressure, cholesterol, and blood sugar
- Stop smoking completely
- Maintain a healthy weight
- Stay physically active
- Seek medical evaluation for symptoms
- Do not ignore changes in chest discomfort

Bridge to the Next Chapter

Now that you understand how blockages form, the next step is to recognize the early warning signal that often appears before a heart attack.

In the next chapter, we will focus on angina — how it feels, how to recognize it, and why it should never be ignored.

CHAPTER 5: Angina — The Early Warning You Should Never Ignore

A Signal Before the Storm

In many patients, the body gives a warning before a heart attack.

That warning is called angina.

In my experience, this is one of the most important opportunities we get in medicine. If recognized early, it can prevent a major event.

But the problem is simple.

Most people do not recognize it.

Or worse, they ignore it.

Angina is not just discomfort. It is the heart asking for attention.

What Angina Really Feels Like

One of the biggest misconceptions is that angina is always severe pain.

In reality, it is often described as:

- Pressure in the chest
- Heaviness or tightness
- A squeezing sensation
- A vague discomfort rather than sharp pain

It is usually felt in the center of the chest, but it may also spread to:

- One or both arms
- Neck or jaw
- Back or shoulders
- Upper abdomen

Some patients notice:

- Shortness of breath
- Fatigue during activity
- Mild sweating

This is why many patients say, “It was not really pain.”

When Angina Occurs

Angina usually appears when the heart needs more oxygen.

Common triggers include:

- Walking or climbing stairs
- Physical exertion
- Emotional stress
- Cold weather
- After heavy meals

When the demand decreases, such as with rest, symptoms often improve.

This pattern is very important.

Stable Angina — Predictable but Serious

Stable angina follows a consistent pattern.

- Occurs with exertion
- Improves with rest
- Remains similar over time

Because it is predictable, many patients begin to ignore it.

That is a mistake.

It indicates significant narrowing in the coronary arteries.

It is a warning that the disease is present.

Unstable Angina — A Dangerous Change

Unstable angina represents a change in the pattern.

- Occurs at rest or with minimal activity
- Becomes more frequent

- Lasts longer
- Does not improve easily

This is a serious condition.

It often means a plaque is unstable and may rupture.

A heart attack may follow.

Unstable angina should be treated as a medical emergency.

Other Types of Angina

There are less common forms of angina.

Variant Angina

- Caused by spasm of the artery
- Often occurs at rest

Microvascular Angina

- Involves small blood vessels
- More common in women
- Symptoms may be less typical

These remind us that heart symptoms can vary.

CHAPTER 5

STABLE vs UNSTABLE ANGINA

STABLE ANGINA

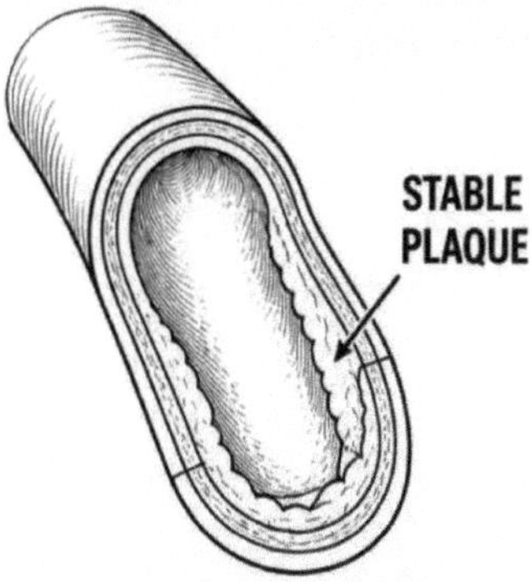

- NARROWING FIXED
- PAIN ON EXERTION RELIEVED BY REST
- PREDICTABLE PATTERN
- OCCURS WITH ACTIVITY

UNSTABLE ANGINA

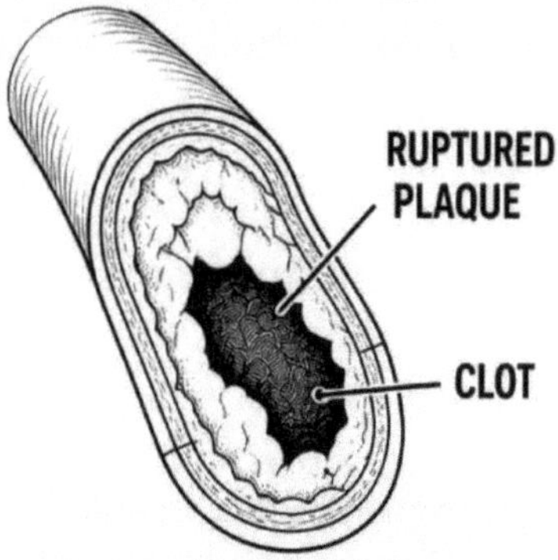

- PLAQUE RUPTURE OR CLOT
- PAIN AT REST OR MINIMAL ACTIVITY
- UNPREDICTABLE SEVERE EPISODES
- HIGH RISK OF HEART ATTACK

TAKEAWAY

UNSTABLE ANGINA IS UNPREDICTABLE AND CAN LEAD TO HEART ATTACK. SEEK MEDICAL CARE IMMEDIATELY.

Angina vs Heart Attack — A Practical Difference

A simple way to understand:

- Angina → reduced blood flow
- Heart attack → blocked blood flow

In angina:

- Symptoms improve with rest or medication

In a heart attack:

- Symptoms persist
- Damage to heart muscle occurs

However, unstable angina and heart attack can appear very similar.

You should never try to distinguish them at home.

A Real-Life Pattern You Should Recognize

A patient feels chest tightness while walking uphill. It improves with rest.

This repeats over several days.

This is typical stable angina.

Later, the same patient feels discomfort at rest. It lasts longer and feels more intense.

This is unstable angina.

If ignored, this can progress to a heart attack.

Doctor's Pearl

A change in the pattern of chest discomfort is often more important than the severity of pain.

Common Mistakes to Avoid

- Ignoring symptoms because they improve with rest
- Continuing activity despite discomfort
- Not seeking evaluation for recurring symptoms
- Assuming mild symptoms are harmless

Red Flag Warnings

Seek urgent medical attention if:

- Chest discomfort occurs at rest
- Symptoms are increasing in frequency
- Pain lasts longer than usual
- Relief is incomplete

- Associated symptoms such as breathlessness or sweating occur

---

Key Points

- Angina is a warning sign of reduced blood flow
- Stable angina is predictable but serious
- Unstable angina is a medical emergency
- Early recognition can prevent a heart attack

Chapter Summary

Angina is an early warning sign that the heart is not receiving enough blood. It is usually felt as pressure, heaviness, or discomfort in the chest, often triggered by activity and relieved by rest. Stable angina follows a predictable pattern, while unstable angina represents a dangerous change that requires urgent attention. Recognizing angina and acting promptly can prevent progression to a heart attack.

Action Plan

- Pay attention to chest discomfort during activity
- Note patterns, triggers, and relief
- Seek medical evaluation for recurring symptoms
- Do not ignore changes in symptoms
- Treat new or worsening symptoms as urgent

Bridge to the Next Chapter

Angina is often a warning.

But what happens when that warning is missed or when a blockage suddenly becomes complete?

In the next chapter, we will understand what happens during a heart attack and why every minute matters.

CHAPTER 6: Heart Attack — What Really Happens Minute by Minute

When a Warning Becomes an Emergency

A heart attack is not just a sudden event. It is the result of a process that has been building for years.

But when it finally occurs, things change very quickly.

Patients often remember the moment clearly.

A discomfort.
A pressure.
A strange feeling that something is not right.

At that moment, inside the body, a critical process has already begun.

A heart attack is injury to the heart muscle caused by loss of blood supply.

Once this begins, time becomes the most important factor.

The First Event — Sudden Blockage

Most heart attacks begin with a sudden event in a coronary artery.

A plaque that has been present for years becomes unstable and ruptures.

When this happens:

- The inner contents of the plaque are exposed
- The body reacts immediately
- A blood clot forms rapidly

This clot can:

- Partially block the artery
- Completely block the artery

When blood flow is reduced or stopped, the heart muscle is at risk.

The First Few Minutes — Oxygen Supply Falls

Within minutes of blockage:

- Blood flow to the heart muscle decreases
- Oxygen supply drops
- Cells begin to function poorly

At this stage, symptoms may begin:

- Chest pressure or heaviness

- Shortness of breath
- A sense of uneasiness

If blood flow is restored quickly, damage can be limited.

---

20 to 40 Minutes — Injury Begins

As the blockage continues:

- Heart muscle cells begin to suffer injury
- The affected area becomes weaker
- The heart's pumping ability may begin to decline

Symptoms often become more noticeable:

- Increasing discomfort
- Sweating
- Nausea
- Fatigue

This is a critical window.

Unfortunately, many patients are still waiting at this stage, hoping symptoms will improve.

---

1 to 2 Hours — Permanent Damage Starts

If blood flow is not restored:

- Irreversible damage to heart muscle begins
- The affected tissue starts to die

At this stage:

- The size of the damage increases with time
- The risk of complications rises

This is why early treatment is so important.

Several Hours — Damage Expands

With continued delay:

- A larger portion of the heart muscle is lost
- The heart becomes weaker
- Recovery becomes more difficult

Complications such as heart failure and abnormal heart rhythms become more likely.

Why "Time Is Muscle"

You will often hear this phrase:

Time is muscle.

It means:

- The sooner blood flow is restored, the more heart muscle is saved
- The longer the delay, the greater the damage

This is not just theory.

It is seen every day in clinical practice.

Different Types of Heart Attack

Not all heart attacks are the same.

STEMI

- Complete blockage of a coronary artery
- More severe
- Requires immediate treatment

NSTEMI

- Partial blockage
- May appear less dramatic
- Still requires urgent care

Both types are serious and require medical attention.

What Happens to the Heart

When part of the heart muscle is damaged:

- That area cannot contract properly
- Overall pumping ability may decrease
- Electrical activity may become unstable

This can lead to:

- Irregular heart rhythms
- Reduced blood flow to the body
- In severe cases, sudden cardiac arrest

Why Outcomes Differ

Not all heart attacks have the same outcome.

The result depends on:

- How quickly treatment begins
- The size of the affected area
- Overall heart health
- Presence of other medical conditions

Early treatment significantly improves survival and recovery.

A Real-Life Comparison

One patient recognizes symptoms early and calls for help.

- Treatment begins quickly
- The artery is opened
- Heart damage is minimal

Another patient delays.

- The blockage continues
- More heart muscle is lost
- Recovery is more difficult

The difference is not chance.

The difference is time.

Doctor's Pearl

Even mild or tolerable chest discomfort can represent a serious heart attack.

Common Mistakes to Avoid

- Waiting for symptoms to become severe
- Assuming discomfort will go away
- Trying home remedies first
- Ignoring associated symptoms
- Delaying medical care

CHAPTER 6

HEART ATTACK

HOW IT HAPPENS

1	2	3	4
PLAQUE RUPTURE	CLOT FORMATION	COMPLETE BLOCKAGE	HEART MUSCLE DAMAGED

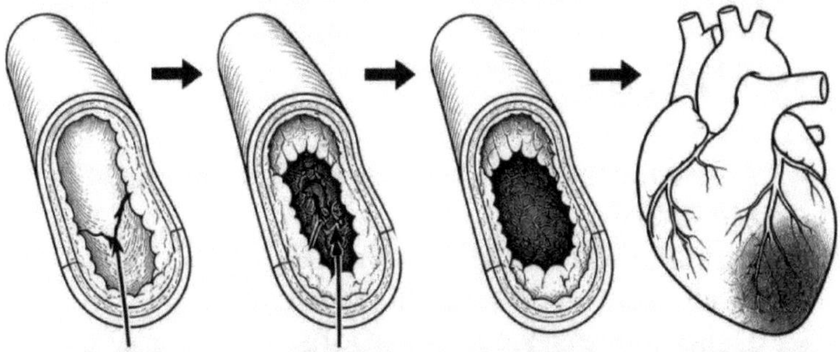

PLAQUE RUPTURES	BLOOD CLOT FORMS	BLOOD FLOW STOPS	HEART MUSCLE BEGINS TO DIE

TIME IS MUSCLE

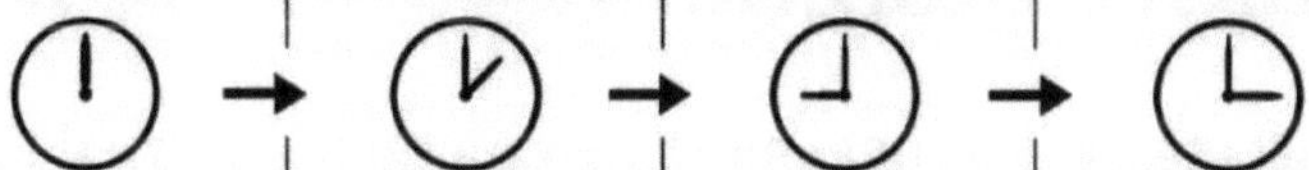

0 MINUTES	20–30 MINUTES	1–2 HOURS	3–6 HOURS
BLOCKAGE OCCURS	HEART MUSCLE BEGINS TO GET DAMAGED	PERMANENT DAMAGE BEGINS	EXTENSIVE MUSCLE DEATH MAY OCCUR

TAKEAWAY

EARLY TREATMENT RESTORES BLOOD FLOW AND SAVES HEART MUSCLE AND LIFE. ACT FAST. EVERY MINUTE COUNTS.

Red Flag Warnings

Seek immediate medical attention if:

- Chest discomfort lasts more than a few minutes
- Symptoms are persistent or worsening
- There is sweating, nausea, or breathlessness
- There is dizziness or unusual weakness

Key Points

- A heart attack is caused by sudden blockage of blood flow
- Damage begins within minutes
- Early treatment saves heart muscle
- Delay increases complications

Chapter Summary

A heart attack is a time-sensitive emergency caused by sudden blockage of blood flow to the heart muscle. Within minutes, the heart begins to suffer, and irreversible damage can occur within hours. The extent of injury depends largely on how quickly treatment is started. Recognizing symptoms early and acting without delay can save heart muscle, preserve heart function, and improve survival.

Action Plan

- Treat persistent chest discomfort as urgent
- Do not wait for symptoms to worsen
- Call emergency services immediately
- Educate family members about warning signs
- Remember that early action saves lives

Bridge to the Next Chapter

Not all heart attacks present in the same way.

In the next chapter, we will explore silent and atypical presentations, especially in women, older adults, and patients with diabetes, where diagnosis is often delayed.

CHAPTER 7: Silent and Atypical Heart Attacks — The Ones People Often Miss

Not Every Heart Attack Looks the Same

When people think of a heart attack, they imagine severe chest pain and sudden collapse.

That does happen.
But in real life, many heart attacks are quieter, less obvious, and easier to miss.

I have seen patients walk into the clinic with nothing more than fatigue or mild discomfort, only to discover that they were having, or had already had, a heart attack.

That is why this chapter is so important.

Not recognizing these subtle presentations is one of the most common reasons for delayed treatment.

What Is a Silent Heart Attack

A silent heart attack is one that:

- Occurs without typical chest pain

- Produces mild or vague symptoms
- Is not recognized at the time

Despite the lack of dramatic symptoms, the heart muscle is still injured.

The danger lies in delay.

Without recognition:

- Medical care is not sought early
- Treatment is delayed
- Damage becomes more extensive

Why Symptoms Can Be Subtle

There are several reasons why symptoms may not be typical.

- The body may not generate strong pain signals
- Nerve function may be altered
- The brain may interpret signals differently
- Other conditions may mask the discomfort

This leads to reduced or altered perception of pain.

Symptoms That Do Not Feel Like a Heart Problem

Instead of classic chest pain, patients may experience:

- Unusual or persistent fatigue
- Shortness of breath
- A feeling of indigestion or discomfort after meals
- Nausea or vomiting
- Pain in the back, neck, jaw, or shoulders
- Lightheadedness or dizziness

These symptoms are often mild.

That is why they are easily ignored.

Heart Attack in Women — Often Different

Women may present differently than men.

While some have typical chest pain, many report:

- Unusual fatigue
- Shortness of breath
- Nausea
- Pain in the upper back or jaw
- A vague sense of discomfort

Because these symptoms are less typical, they are sometimes dismissed or misinterpreted.

Heart Attack in Older Adults — Subtle and Quiet

In older adults, symptoms may be less obvious.

They may include:

- General weakness
- Reduced activity
- Confusion
- Breathlessness

Chest pain may be minimal or absent.

This can delay diagnosis and treatment.

Heart Attack in Patients with Diabetes

Diabetes can affect nerve function.

This may reduce the sensation of pain.

As a result:

- Chest pain may be absent
- Symptoms may be vague
- The first sign may be complications

This makes early recognition more difficult.

Why These Cases Are Missed

There are common reasons:

- Symptoms are mild
- There is no chest pain
- Symptoms are attributed to acidity, fatigue, or stress
- Patients delay seeking care

By the time medical help is sought, damage may already be significant.

A Real-Life Example

A woman in her 50s feels unusually tired for several days. She also notices mild nausea and discomfort in the back.

She assumes it is stress and continues her routine.

Later, when symptoms worsen, she seeks medical care.

Tests show that she had a heart attack.

If the early symptoms had been recognized, treatment could have been started sooner.

Doctor's Pearl

Absence of chest pain does not rule out a heart attack.

CHAPTER 7

TYPES OF HEART ATTACK

MAIN CATEGORIES

1 STEMI
(COMPLETE BLOCKAGE)

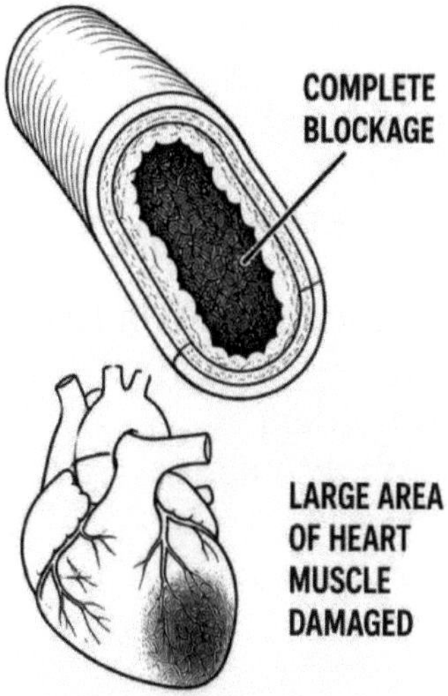

SEVERE CHEST PAIN
LONGER DURATION
HIGHER RISK

2 NSTEMI
(PARTIAL BLOCKAGE)

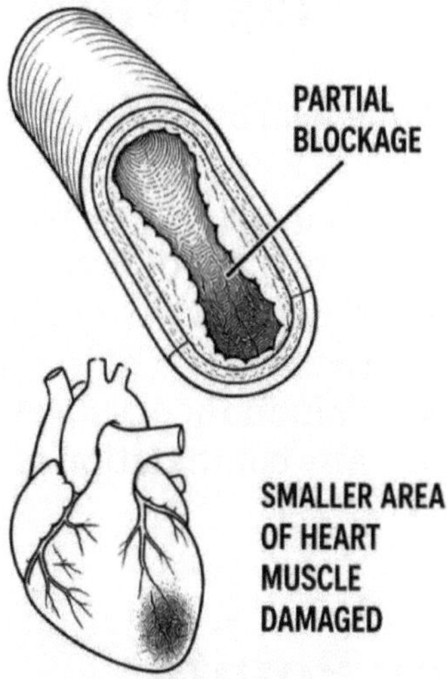

CHEST PAIN MAY BE
LESS SEVERE
RISK STILL PRESENT

TAKEAWAY

BOTH TYPES ARE SERIOUS.
EARLY RECOGNITION AND TREATMENT
IMPROVE OUTCOMES AND SAVE LIVES.

Common Mistakes to Avoid

- Ignoring unexplained fatigue
- Assuming symptoms are due to acidity or stress
- Delaying medical evaluation
- Not recognizing atypical symptoms

Red Flag Warnings

Seek medical attention if you experience:

- Unusual fatigue without clear cause
- Shortness of breath
- Nausea or discomfort not explained by routine causes
- Pain in the back, jaw, or shoulders
- Any combination of these symptoms

Key Points

- Not all heart attacks present with chest pain
- Women, older adults, and patients with diabetes often have atypical symptoms
- Silent heart attacks can still cause serious damage
- Early recognition is essential

Chapter Summary

Silent and atypical heart attacks are more common than many people realize. They often present with mild or unusual symptoms such as fatigue, breathlessness, or indigestion rather than classic chest pain. Women, older adults, and patients with diabetes are more likely to have these presentations. Because these symptoms are easily misinterpreted, diagnosis is often delayed, leading to greater heart damage. Awareness of these patterns is essential for early detection and timely treatment.

Action Plan

- Pay attention to unexplained or unusual symptoms
- Do not ignore persistent fatigue or breathlessness
- Seek medical evaluation early
- Be especially cautious if you have diabetes or other risk factors
- Educate your family about atypical symptoms

Bridge to the Next Chapter

Now that you understand how heart attacks can present in different ways, the next important step is to understand why these problems develop in the first place.

In the next chapter, we will focus on the risk factors that quietly damage the heart over time and how you can take control of them.

CHAPTER 8: Risk Factors That Quietly Damage the Heart — What You Can Change and What You Cannot

The Disease Begins Long Before Symptoms

By the time chest pain appears, the disease is often already well established.

This is one of the most important truths in heart care.

Coronary artery disease develops silently over many years.

During this silent phase, risk factors are at work.

They slowly damage blood vessels, promote plaque formation, and increase the likelihood of future heart events.

The encouraging part is this:

Many of these risk factors are under your control.

Two Types of Risk Factors

To understand risk clearly, divide factors into two groups.

Non-modifiable Risk Factors

These are factors you cannot change:

- Age
- Family history
- Biological sex

These determine your baseline risk.

Modifiable Risk Factors

These are the factors you can control:

- High blood pressure
- Diabetes
- High cholesterol
- Smoking
- Excess body weight
- Physical inactivity
- Unhealthy diet
- Poor sleep
- Chronic stress

This is where your greatest opportunity lies.

High Blood Pressure — The Silent Damage

High blood pressure damages the inner lining of arteries.

Over time:

- Arteries become stiff
- Plaque forms more easily
- The heart works harder

Most patients feel no symptoms.

That is why regular monitoring is essential.

Diabetes — A Powerful Risk Multiplier

Diabetes significantly increases the risk of heart disease.

High blood sugar:

- Damages blood vessels
- Promotes inflammation
- Accelerates plaque buildup

It also affects nerve function, which can reduce pain sensation and lead to silent heart attacks.

Proper control is critical.

CHAPTER 8

RISK FACTORS

FOR HEART DISEASE AND HEART ATTACK

1. **HIGH BLOOD PRESSURE**

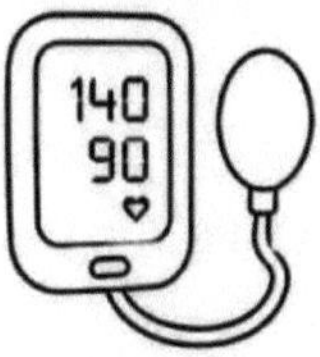

2. **HIGH CHOLESTEROL**

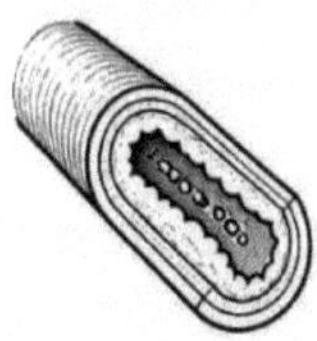

3. **DIABETES**

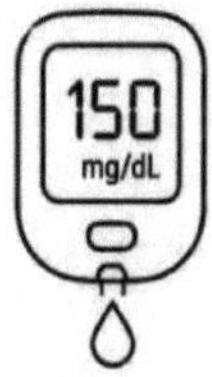

4. **SMOKING**

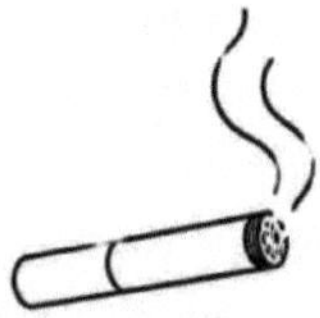

5. **OBESITY**

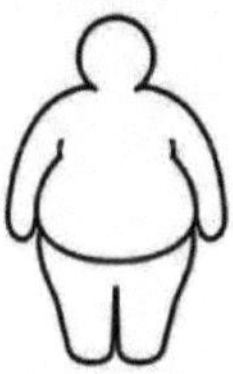

6. **PHYSICAL INACTIVITY**

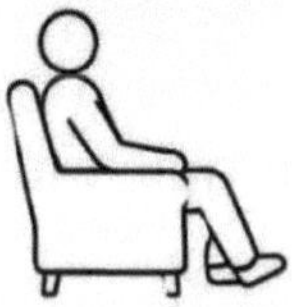

7. **UNHEALTHY DIET**

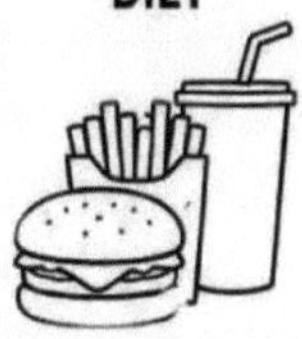

8. **STRESS**

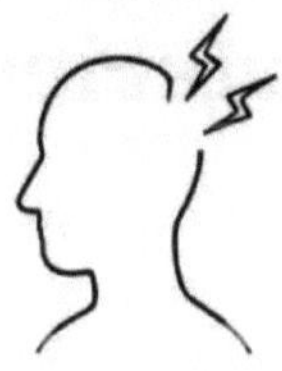

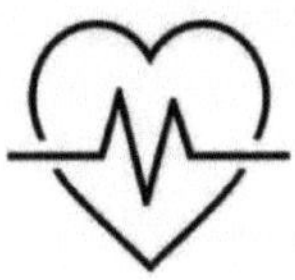

TAKEAWAY

MANY RISK FACTORS CAN BE CONTROLLED. HEALTHY LIFESTYLE, EARLY DETECTION, AND PROPER MANAGEMENT CAN PREVENT HEART DISEASE AND HEART ATTACK.

Cholesterol — The Building Material of Plaque

Cholesterol plays a central role in artery blockage.

- LDL contributes to plaque formation
- HDL helps remove excess cholesterol

When LDL levels are high:

- Plaque builds more easily
- Arteries narrow faster
- Risk of heart attack increases

Managing cholesterol is one of the most effective preventive steps.

Smoking — Direct Injury to the Arteries

Smoking affects the heart in multiple ways.

It:

- Damages the inner lining of blood vessels
- Promotes clot formation
- Reduces oxygen supply
- Increases heart rate and blood pressure

There is no safe level of smoking.

Stopping smoking is one of the most powerful steps you can take.

Excess Weight and Physical Inactivity

These two factors often occur together.

They contribute to:

- High blood pressure
- Poor blood sugar control
- Abnormal cholesterol
- Increased inflammation

Even modest weight loss and regular physical activity can produce significant benefits.

Diet — Daily Choices That Matter

Diet is not about perfection.

It is about consistent patterns.

A heart-healthy diet includes:

- Fruits and vegetables
- Whole grains
- Nuts and seeds
- Healthy oils

- Lean protein sources

It limits:

- Processed foods
- Sugary drinks
- Excess salt
- Saturated and trans fats

Small changes, maintained over time, create lasting results.

Sleep — Often Ignored but Essential

Poor sleep has a direct impact on heart health.

It can:

- Raise blood pressure
- Affect blood sugar
- Increase appetite
- Worsen stress

Most adults need about 7 to 8 hours of quality sleep.

If sleep is poor or interrupted, it should be evaluated.

Stress — The Hidden Contributor

Chronic stress affects the heart in subtle but important ways.

It can:

- Raise blood pressure
- Affect heart rhythm
- Lead to unhealthy habits

Managing stress is not about eliminating it, but learning to respond to it more effectively.

Family History and Age — Not Under Your Control

Some factors cannot be changed.

Risk increases with age, and a strong family history increases susceptibility.

But this does not mean you are powerless.

Controlling modifiable risk factors can significantly reduce overall risk.

A Simple Way to Understand Risk

I often explain it like this:

Your genes may increase your risk, but your lifestyle determines how that risk develops.

Doctor's Pearl

The more risk factors you control, the more you reduce your overall risk.

Common Mistakes to Avoid

- Ignoring borderline abnormal values
- Not monitoring blood pressure or blood sugar
- Continuing smoking
- Relying only on medications without lifestyle change
- Neglecting sleep and stress

Red Flag Warnings

Pay attention if:

- Blood pressure remains elevated

- Blood sugar is poorly controlled
- Cholesterol levels are high
- Weight is increasing
- Physical activity is decreasing

These are early warning signs.

Key Points

- Risk factors act silently over time
- Many important factors are controllable
- Early control prevents serious disease
- Lifestyle and medical care must work together

Chapter Summary

Coronary artery disease develops over time due to a combination of risk factors. While some factors such as age and family history cannot be changed, many others are within your control. Managing blood pressure, blood sugar, cholesterol, and lifestyle habits can significantly reduce the risk of angina and heart attack. Prevention begins long before symptoms appear.

Action Plan

- Monitor blood pressure regularly
- Check blood sugar and cholesterol

- Stop smoking completely
- Maintain a healthy weight
- Stay physically active
- Follow a balanced diet
- Improve sleep and manage stress

Bridge to the Next Chapter

Now that you understand the risk factors behind heart disease, the next important step is to recognize that not all chest pain comes from the heart.

In the next chapter, we will explore other causes of chest pain and how to tell them apart.

CHAPTER 9: Other Causes of Chest Pain — Not Everything Is the Heart, But Some Things Still Matter

A Calm and Balanced Approach

By now, you understand how important chest pain can be.

But there is another equally important truth:

Not all chest pain is caused by the heart.

In fact, many people who come to the emergency room with chest discomfort do not have a heart attack.

That is reassuring.

But here is the part that requires judgment:

Some non-heart causes can still be serious.

So the goal is not to panic, and not to ignore.

The goal is to think clearly and act wisely.

Where Can Chest Pain Come From

The chest contains several structures.

Pain can arise from:

- The heart
- The esophagus and stomach
- The lungs
- The muscles and ribs
- The major blood vessels
- Emotional or stress-related causes

Because these structures are close to each other, their symptoms can overlap.

This is why chest pain can be confusing.

Acid Reflux — The Most Common Cause

Acid reflux is one of the most frequent causes of chest discomfort.

It is often described as:

- A burning sensation behind the breastbone
- Pain after meals
- Discomfort that worsens when lying down

It may improve with antacids.

But an important point must be remembered:

Heart-related pain can sometimes feel very similar.

Never assume new or unusual chest discomfort is just acidity, especially if it is different from your usual pattern.

Muscle and Rib Pain — Often Localized

Pain from the chest wall is usually easier to recognize.

It is often:

- Sharp or localized
- Worse with movement
- Worse with deep breathing
- Reproducible with pressure on the area

This type of pain is usually less serious.

But its location in the chest often causes concern.

Lung-Related Causes — Sometimes Serious

Certain lung conditions can cause chest pain and require prompt attention.

Pulmonary Embolism

- A blood clot in the lung
- Sudden chest pain
- Shortness of breath
- May occur after prolonged immobility or travel

Pneumonia

- Infection in the lung
- Chest pain with fever and cough
- Pain may worsen with breathing

Pneumothorax

- Collapse of part of the lung
- Sudden sharp chest pain
- Breathlessness

These conditions require medical evaluation.

Aortic Problems — Rare but Dangerous

One important but less common condition is aortic dissection.

It is often described as:

- Sudden severe pain
- A tearing sensation
- Pain radiating to the back

This is a medical emergency and requires immediate care.

Anxiety and Panic — Real Symptoms

Emotional stress can produce physical symptoms.

Patients may experience:

- Chest tightness
- Rapid heartbeat
- Shortness of breath
- A feeling of fear

These symptoms can closely mimic a heart attack.

Even when anxiety is suspected, heart causes must be ruled out first.

How Doctors Tell the Difference

Doctors do not rely on a single feature.

They evaluate:

- The nature of the pain
- Duration and pattern
- Associated symptoms
- Risk factors
- Physical examination
- Diagnostic tests

They ask questions such as:

- When did it start
- What triggers it
- What relieves it
- Has it changed over time

This structured approach helps reach a safe diagnosis.

A Practical Comparison

Two patients may describe chest discomfort.

One has burning pain after meals, improves with antacids, and has no major risk factors.

Another has pressure during activity, sweating, and breathlessness.

The first is more likely to have reflux.

The second raises concern for heart disease.

Context is everything.

Doctor's Pearl

When chest pain is new, unusual, or associated with risk factors, it should always be evaluated as a possible heart problem first.

Common Mistakes to Avoid

- Assuming all chest pain is acidity
- Ignoring mild symptoms
- Self-diagnosing without evaluation
- Delaying medical care
- Overlooking serious non-heart causes

Red Flag Warnings

Seek medical attention if chest pain is associated with:

- Shortness of breath
- Sudden onset and severe intensity
- Pain spreading to the back or arm
- Dizziness or fainting
- Fever with chest discomfort

CHAPTER 9

SIGNS AND SYMPTOMS

OF HEART ATTACK

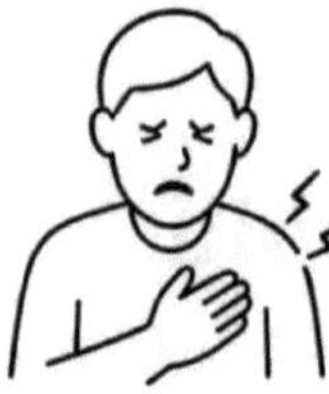

1. CHEST PAIN
(PRESSURE, TIGHTNESS OR DISCOMFORT)

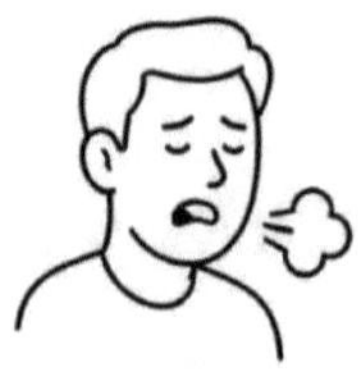

2. SHORTNESS OF BREATH

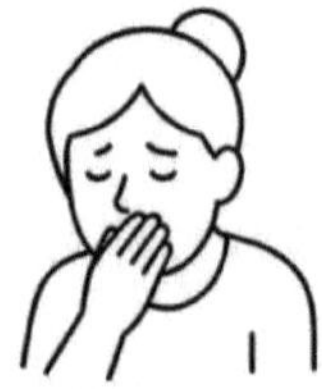

3. NAUSEA OR VOMITING

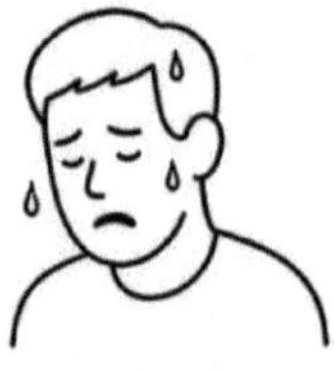

4. COLD SWEAT

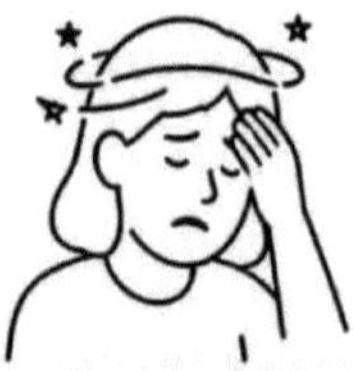

5. DIZZINESS
OR LIGHTHEADEDNESS

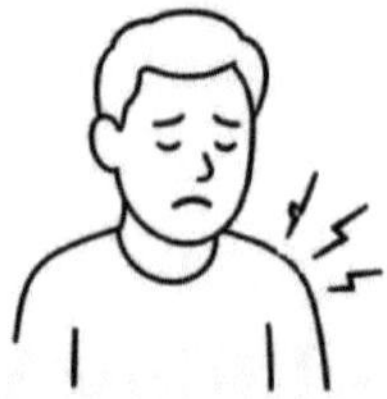

6. PAIN RADIATING
TO ARM, SHOULDER, NECK, JAW OR BACK

SYMPTOMS MAY VARY.
SOME PEOPLE MAY NOT HAVE ALL THESE SIGNS.

TAKEAWAY

RECOGNIZING SYMPTOMS EARLY AND SEEKING IMMEDIATE MEDICAL HELP CAN SAVE LIVES.

Key Points

- Chest pain can arise from multiple causes
- Not all chest pain is heart-related
- Some non-heart causes can still be serious
- Proper evaluation is essential

Chapter Summary

Chest pain is not always caused by the heart. It may originate from the digestive system, lungs, chest wall, or even emotional stress. While many of these causes are less serious, some can be life-threatening. Because symptoms often overlap, it is important to evaluate new or unusual chest pain carefully. A balanced approach helps avoid both unnecessary fear and dangerous delay.

Action Plan

- Do not assume the cause of chest pain
- Pay attention to patterns and associated symptoms
- Seek medical evaluation when symptoms are new or unclear
- Treat chest pain seriously until proven otherwise
- Follow medical advice for further testing if needed

Bridge to the Next Chapter

Now that you understand the possible causes of chest pain, the next important step is to understand how doctors evaluate it.

In the next chapter, we will walk through what happens when you seek medical care and how doctors decide what to do next.

CHAPTER 10: How Doctors Evaluate Chest Pain — What Really Happens When You Seek Care

From Uncertainty to Clarity

When you arrive at a clinic or emergency room with chest pain, things can feel fast and overwhelming.

Monitors are attached.
Questions come quickly.
Tests are ordered.

Behind all this activity, there is a clear and careful thought process.

Every doctor is trying to answer one critical question:

Is this a life-threatening condition, or something less dangerous?

This decision must be made quickly, but also safely.

Your Story — The Most Important Step

Before any test is done, your doctor begins with your history.

This is often the most important part of the evaluation.

You may be asked:

- When did the discomfort start
- What does it feel like
- Where is it located
- What brings it on
- What makes it better or worse
- Has it changed over time

Certain patterns immediately raise concern:

- Pressure or heaviness in the chest
- Symptoms during exertion
- Pain lasting several minutes
- Associated sweating or breathlessness

On the other hand, sharp pain that changes with movement may suggest a non-heart cause.

Your description guides the entire evaluation.

Understanding Your Risk

Symptoms alone are not enough.

Your background plays an important role.

Doctors consider:

- Age
- Blood pressure

- Diabetes
- Cholesterol
- Smoking history
- Family history

A person with multiple risk factors is evaluated very differently from someone with none.

This is called risk assessment.

Vital Signs and Physical Examination

Next comes a focused examination.

This includes checking:

- Blood pressure
- Heart rate
- Oxygen level
- Temperature

The doctor listens to your heart and lungs and looks for:

- Signs of heart failure
- Lung conditions
- Chest wall tenderness

While the exam alone may not give a diagnosis, it provides valuable clues.

CHAPTER 10

DIAGNOSIS OF HEART DISEASE

COMMON TESTS

1. ECG

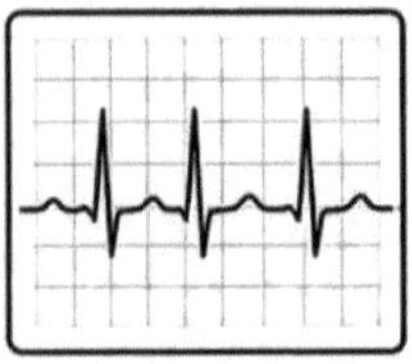

CHECKS HEART RHYTHM

2. ECHOCARDIOGRAM

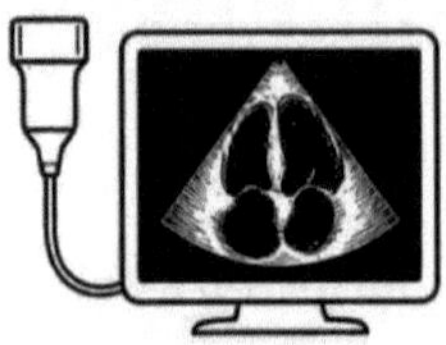

ASSESSS HEART STRUCTURE AND FUNCTION

3. TREADMILL TEST

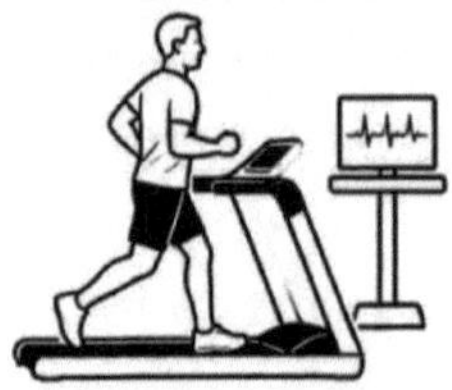

EVALUATES HEART RESPONSE TO EXERCISE

4. BLOOD TESTS

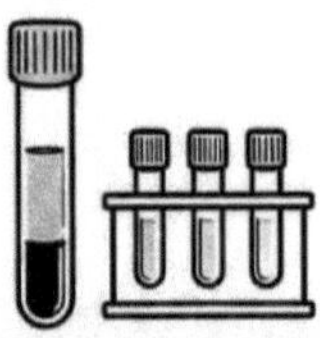

CHECKS CHOLESTEROL, SUGAR AND OTHER RISK FACTORS

5. STRESS IMAGING

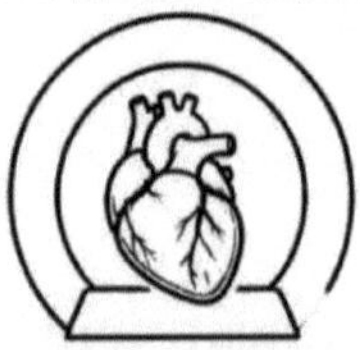

DETECTS REDUCED BLOOD FLOW

6. CORONARY ANGIOGRAPHY

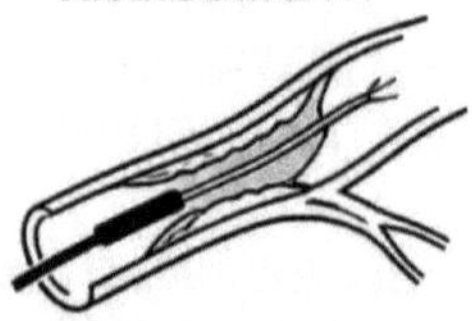

IDENTIFIES BLOCKAGES IN CORONARY ARTERIES

EARLY AND ACCURATE DIAGNOSIS LEADS TO BETTER TREATMENT AND OUTCOMES.

TAKEAWAY

APPROPRIATE TESTS HELP FIND THE CAUSE, ASSESS SEVERITY, AND GUIDE TREATMENT FOR HEART DISEASE.

Deciding the Level of Risk

One of the most important steps is classifying the level of risk.

Patients are broadly grouped into:

- High risk
- Intermediate risk
- Low risk

High Risk Features

- Ongoing chest discomfort
- Typical heart-related symptoms
- Abnormal vital signs
- Significant risk factors

These patients require urgent care.

Low Risk Features

- Atypical symptoms
- Stable condition
- No major risk factors

These patients may be evaluated more gradually.

Emergency Room vs Office Evaluation

Where you are evaluated depends on your risk.

Emergency Room

- Rapid assessment
- Immediate testing
- Continuous monitoring

Doctor's Office

- Suitable for stable, low-risk cases
- Allows detailed discussion
- Focus on long-term care

If there is any doubt, emergency evaluation is the safer choice.

Why Observation May Be Needed

Patients often ask:

"If my initial tests are normal, why do I need to stay?"

The reason is simple.

Early tests may not detect all problems.

Doctors may recommend observation because:

- Symptoms can evolve
- Blood test changes may take time
- Repeat evaluation improves accuracy

This approach increases safety.

Why Some Patients Are Sent Home

Patients may be discharged if:

- Their risk is low
- Initial evaluation is reassuring
- Symptoms are not suggestive of serious disease

However, discharge is not the end of care.

It usually includes:

- Follow-up testing
- Monitoring of symptoms
- Risk factor management

A Real-Life Comparison

Two patients present with chest discomfort.

One has pressure during exertion, sweating, and diabetes.

This patient is treated as high risk.

Another has sharp pain that worsens with movement and has no risk factors.

This patient is likely low risk.

The difference is not just the symptom.

It is the overall clinical picture.

Doctor's Pearl

In chest pain evaluation, the combination of symptoms and risk factors is more important than any single test.

Common Mistakes to Avoid

- Ignoring symptoms because they seem mild
- Assuming a normal exam means no heart problem
- Not sharing complete information
- Delaying medical evaluation
- Skipping follow-up

Red Flag Warnings

Immediate attention is required if:

- Chest pain is ongoing
- Symptoms are worsening
- Significant risk factors are present
- Associated symptoms such as breathlessness or sweating occur

---

Key Points

- Chest pain evaluation follows a structured approach
- History and risk factors are critical
- Patients are categorized based on risk
- Decisions are based on the full clinical picture

Chapter Summary

When you seek care for chest pain, doctors follow a systematic approach to determine the cause and urgency. The evaluation begins with your history and risk factors, followed by examination and early testing. Based on this information, patients are classified into risk categories, which guide further management. This structured method helps identify serious conditions quickly while avoiding unnecessary interventions.

Action Plan

- Provide clear and complete information about your symptoms
- Know your personal risk factors
- Seek medical care without delay when needed
- Follow all medical advice
- Complete recommended follow-up

Bridge to the Next Chapter

Now that you understand how doctors evaluate chest pain, the next step is to understand the tests they use.

In the next chapter, we will explain common heart tests in simple language so you know what they show and why they are done.

CHAPTER 11: Heart Tests Explained — What They Show, What They Don't, and Why They Matter

From Symptoms to Clear Answers

After the initial evaluation, your doctor may recommend tests.

At this stage, many patients feel uncertain.

They ask:

- "Why do I need so many tests?"
- "If one test is normal, does that mean I am fine?"
- "What exactly are these tests looking for?"

These are very reasonable questions.

Let me simplify this clearly.

No single test gives the full answer.

Each test looks at a different aspect of the heart.
Together, they help form a complete and reliable picture.

Electrocardiogram (ECG) — The First Step

An ECG records the electrical activity of your heart.

It is:

- Quick
- Painless
- Widely available

It can detect:

- Ongoing heart attack
- Previous heart damage
- Abnormal heart rhythms

But it has an important limitation.

A normal ECG does not rule out heart disease.

That is why further evaluation is often needed.

Troponin Blood Test — Detecting Heart Muscle Injury

Troponin is a blood test that detects damage to the heart muscle.

When heart cells are injured, troponin levels rise.

This test helps:

- Confirm a heart attack
- Detect even small amounts of damage

However:

- Troponin may take a few hours to rise

For this reason, the test is often repeated.

A single normal result early on does not always mean everything is normal.

Echocardiogram — Seeing the Heart in Motion

An echocardiogram is an ultrasound of the heart.

It shows:

- Heart chambers
- Heart valves
- Pumping function

It can detect:

- Areas of reduced movement
- Effects of previous heart damage
- Structural abnormalities

It is safe and painless.

Stress Test — Evaluating the Heart Under Load

A stress test evaluates how your heart performs when it needs more oxygen.

This is done by:

- Walking on a treadmill
- Or using medication if exercise is not possible

During the test:

- ECG is monitored
- Symptoms are assessed

Sometimes imaging is added to improve accuracy.

This test helps detect:

- Reduced blood flow during activity
- Possible blockages

CT Calcium Score — Detecting Early Risk

This scan measures calcium deposits in the coronary arteries.

It helps:

- Detect early plaque
- Estimate long-term risk

It is useful for prevention in people without symptoms.

However:

- It does not show exact blockage severity
- It is not used in emergency situations

Coronary CT Angiography — A Detailed Non-Invasive Test

This test provides detailed images of the coronary arteries.

It can show:

- Narrowing of arteries
- Location of plaque
- Overall structure

It is non-invasive and increasingly used in modern practice.

Coronary Angiogram — The Most Accurate Test

A coronary angiogram is the gold standard for detecting blockages.

It involves:

- Inserting a catheter through a blood vessel
- Injecting contrast dye
- Taking detailed images of the arteries

It shows:

- Exact location and severity of blockages

It also allows immediate treatment such as angioplasty and stenting.

Because it is invasive, it is used when clearly needed.

Why More Than One Test Is Needed

Patients often wonder why multiple tests are recommended.

The reason is simple.

Each test answers a different question:

- ECG → electrical activity
- Troponin → muscle injury
- Stress test → function under stress
- Angiogram → anatomy

Together, they provide a complete understanding.

A Real-Life Example

A patient presents with chest discomfort.

- ECG is normal
- Initial troponin is normal

But symptoms continue.

Further testing reveals a significant blockage.

This is why relying on a single test can be misleading.

Doctor's Pearl

A normal test result does not always mean a normal heart. Clinical judgment and follow-up are essential.

Common Mistakes to Avoid

- Assuming one normal test rules out heart disease
- Avoiding recommended tests due to fear
- Not completing follow-up testing
- Misunderstanding test results

Red Flag Warnings

Further evaluation is needed if:

- Symptoms persist
- Risk factors are present
- Symptoms worsen
- There is uncertainty about diagnosis

Key Points

- Different tests evaluate different aspects of heart health
- No single test provides all answers
- Some tests detect damage, others detect risk
- Proper interpretation requires medical expertise

Chapter Summary

Heart tests are essential tools in diagnosing and managing chest pain and coronary artery disease. Each test provides specific information, whether it is electrical activity, heart muscle injury, function, or anatomy. Understanding these tests helps reduce anxiety and allows you to participate actively in your care. A combination of tests, along with clinical judgment, ensures accurate diagnosis and appropriate treatment.

Action Plan

- Understand why each test is recommended
- Do not delay or skip necessary tests
- Follow instructions carefully before testing
- Discuss results clearly with your doctor
- Ask questions if anything is unclear

Bridge to the Next Chapter

Now that you understand how heart problems are diagnosed, the next step is treatment.

In the next chapter, we will discuss what happens during emergency treatment of a heart attack and how timely care can save your life.

CHAPTER 12: Emergency Treatment of a Heart Attack — What Happens When Every Minute Counts

From Suspicion to Immediate Action

Once a heart attack is suspected, everything changes.

There is no time to wait.
No time to observe.
No time to take chances.

The goal becomes very clear:

Restore blood flow to the heart as quickly as possible.

Modern treatment has made remarkable progress. Many patients today survive and recover well because care begins early.

But one truth remains unchanged:

The outcome depends greatly on how quickly treatment begins.

What Happens When You Reach the Hospital

The moment you arrive, a coordinated process begins.

You are:

- Placed on a heart monitor
- Evaluated rapidly
- Given an ECG within minutes
- Sent for urgent blood tests

At the same time, treatment may begin immediately.

Doctors do not always wait for every test result when suspicion is high.

Because in a heart attack:

Speed matters more than delay for certainty.

Aspirin — A Simple but Powerful First Step

One of the first medications given is aspirin.

It works by:

- Reducing the ability of platelets to form clots
- Slowing the progression of blockage

This simple step can improve survival.

If previously advised by your doctor, chewing aspirin at the onset of symptoms may help, unless there is a contraindication.

Nitroglycerin — Reducing the Heart's Workload

Nitroglycerin is often given under the tongue.

It helps:

- Relax blood vessels
- Reduce the heart's workload
- Improve blood flow

It may relieve symptoms, but it does not remove the blockage.

Blood Thinners — Stabilizing the Situation

Additional medications are used to prevent the clot from growing.

These include:

- Antiplatelet drugs

- Anticoagulants

They help:

- Stabilize the blockage
- Reduce further clot formation
- Prepare the patient for definitive treatment

Pain Relief and Monitoring

Pain and anxiety increase the workload on the heart.

Managing these is important.

This includes:

- Pain relief medications
- Continuous monitoring
- Supportive care

These steps help reduce stress on the heart during a critical period.

The Most Important Step — Opening the Blocked Artery

The key treatment in a heart attack is restoring blood flow.

There are two main approaches.

Primary Angioplasty — The Preferred Method

This is the most effective treatment in many cases.

A catheter is inserted through a blood vessel and guided to the blocked artery.

At the site of blockage:

- A balloon is inflated
- The artery is opened
- A stent is placed to keep it open

This restores blood flow quickly and effectively.

Clot-Dissolving Medications

If angioplasty is not immediately available, clot-dissolving drugs may be used.

These medications:

- Break down the clot
- Restore blood flow

They are most effective when given early.

Why Timing Makes All the Difference

The earlier the artery is opened:

- The more heart muscle is saved
- The better the recovery
- The lower the risk of complications

Delay leads to:

- Greater damage
- Reduced heart function
- Increased long-term problems

What Happens After Blood Flow Is Restored

Once the artery is opened:

- Symptoms usually improve
- Heart function is assessed
- Further treatment is planned

You will be monitored for:

- Heart rhythm abnormalities
- Blood pressure changes
- Signs of complications

This phase is essential for stabilization.

A Real-Life Comparison

One patient reaches the hospital early.

- Treatment begins quickly
- Blood flow is restored
- Heart damage is minimal

Another patient delays.

- The blockage persists longer
- More heart muscle is lost
- Recovery becomes difficult

Once again, the difference is timing.

Doctor's Pearl

The most effective treatment for a heart attack is early treatment.

Common Mistakes to Avoid

- Delaying hospital arrival
- Ignoring early symptoms
- Trying home remedies first
- Underestimating the seriousness of symptoms

Red Flag Warnings

Seek immediate emergency care if:

- Chest discomfort persists
- Symptoms worsen
- There is shortness of breath or sweating
- There is dizziness or fainting

Key Points

- Emergency treatment focuses on restoring blood flow
- Aspirin and blood thinners are critical early steps
- Angioplasty is the preferred treatment when available
- Early action improves survival

Chapter Summary

Emergency treatment of a heart attack focuses on quickly restoring blood flow to the heart muscle. Initial care includes medications such as aspirin, nitroglycerin, and blood thinners, followed by definitive treatment with angioplasty or clot-dissolving drugs. The sooner treatment begins, the better the chances of survival and recovery. Understanding this process reinforces the importance of acting quickly when symptoms occur.

Action Plan

- Recognize symptoms early
- Call emergency services immediately
- Do not delay seeking care
- Follow medical advice promptly
- Remember that early treatment saves lives

Bridge to the Next Chapter

Once the emergency phase is over, treatment does not stop.

In the next chapter, we will discuss the medications that protect your heart long term and reduce the risk of future heart problems.

CHAPTER 13: Medicines That Protect Your Heart — The Treatment That Works Quietly Every Day

The Moment Many Patients Let Their Guard Down

After a heart attack or a procedure like a stent, many patients feel relieved.

The pain is gone.
The emergency has passed.
Life begins to feel normal again.

This feeling is natural.

But this is also the moment when many patients make a serious mistake.

They begin to think:

"Now I am cured."

The reality is different.

The treatment is not over. In many ways, it has just begun.

HOW HEART DISEASE IS TREATED

Treatment aims to relieve symptoms, improve quality of life, and reduce risk of heart attack and complications.

1. LIFESTYLE CHANGES

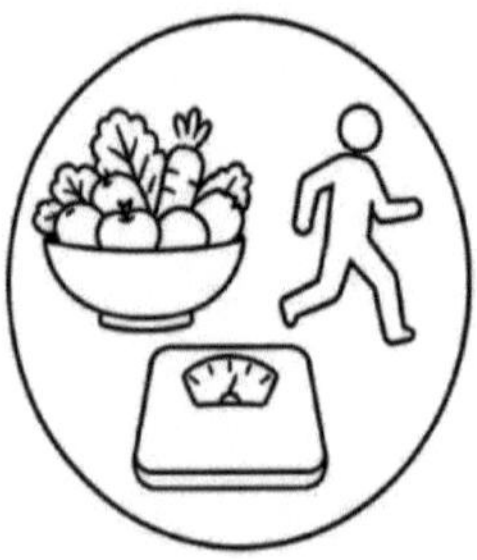

Healthy diet, regular exercise, maintain healthy weight, stop smoking, manage stress.

2. MEDICINES

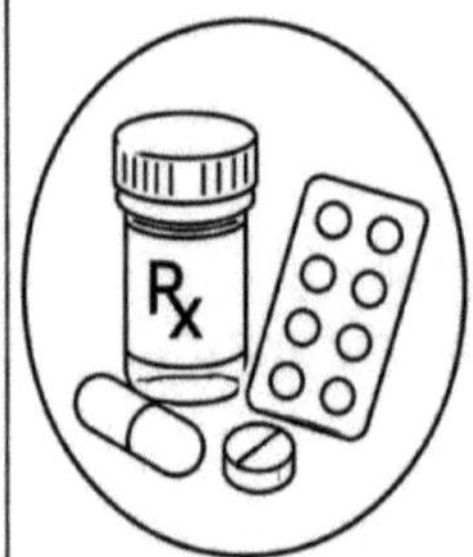

Medications to control blood pressure, cholesterol, diabetes, and prevent blood clots.

3. PROCEDURES & SURGERY

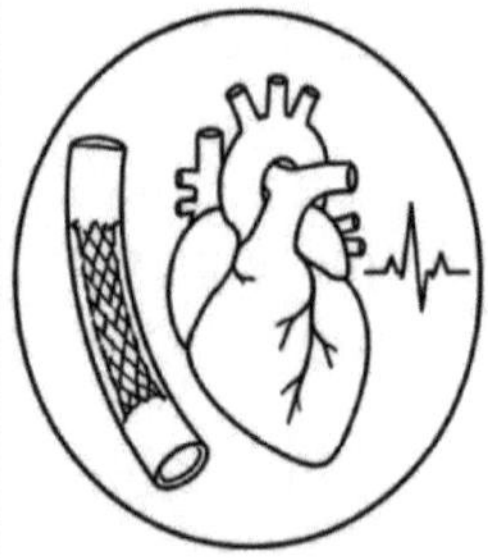

Angioplasty with stent, bypass surgery, and other procedures to restore blood flow.

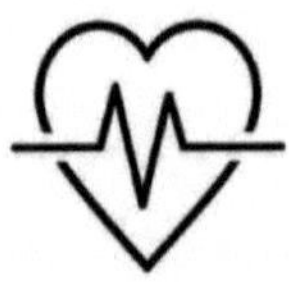

TAKEAWAY

The right combination of lifestyle changes, medicines, and procedures can improve heart health and help you live a longer, healthier life.

Why Medicines Remain Essential

Even after successful treatment:

- The underlying disease is still present
- Plaque may exist in other arteries
- Risk factors may still be active

Medicines are not just for symptom relief.

They are for **protection**.

They help:

- Prevent clot formation
- Stabilize plaque
- Reduce strain on the heart
- Lower the risk of future heart events

You may not feel their effect, but they are working continuously.

Antiplatelet Medicines — Preventing Dangerous Clots

These are among the most important medications.

They reduce the ability of platelets to stick together and form clots.

Common examples include:

- Aspirin
- Additional antiplatelet medications as prescribed

These are especially critical after stent placement.

Stopping them suddenly can lead to clot formation within the stent, which can be life-threatening.

Statins — More Than Just Cholesterol Control

Statins are a cornerstone of heart protection.

They:

- Lower LDL cholesterol
- Reduce inflammation in artery walls
- Stabilize plaque

Even patients with normal cholesterol levels may benefit, because these medicines protect the arteries in multiple ways.

Beta Blockers — Reducing the Heart's Workload

Beta blockers help the heart work more efficiently.

They:

- Slow the heart rate
- Lower blood pressure
- Reduce oxygen demand

This reduces strain on the heart and improves long-term outcomes.

ACE Inhibitors and ARBs — Protecting the Heart and Blood Vessels

These medications:

- Lower blood pressure
- Improve blood vessel function
- Reduce strain on the heart

They are particularly useful in patients with:

- High blood pressure
- Diabetes
- Reduced heart function

Nitrates and Anti-Anginal Medicines — Relieving Symptoms

These medications help relieve chest discomfort.

They:

- Improve blood flow
- Reduce the workload on the heart

They are often used in patients with angina.

Additional Medications — Tailored to You

Depending on your condition, your doctor may prescribe:

- Additional blood thinners
- Advanced cholesterol-lowering medications
- Diabetes medications
- Drugs to control heart rhythm

Treatment is always individualized.

The Most Important Rule — Take Them Regularly

One of the most common and dangerous problems I see is this:

Patients stop taking medicines when they feel better.

This can lead to:

- Increased risk of clot formation
- Recurrence of symptoms
- Another heart attack

These medicines protect you every day, even when you feel completely fine.

Understanding Side Effects Without Fear

All medications can have side effects.

However:

- Most side effects are mild
- Serious side effects are uncommon
- Alternatives are often available

The key is communication.

Never stop a medication on your own. Always discuss concerns with your doctor.

A Real-Life Perspective

One patient takes medications regularly, follows advice, and attends follow-up visits.

Years later, he remains stable.

Another patient stops medications after feeling better.

Within months, he returns with another heart problem.

The difference is not chance.

The difference is consistency.

Doctor's Pearl

Medicines after a heart event are not optional. They are your long-term protection.

Common Mistakes to Avoid

- Stopping medications when you feel better
- Missing doses frequently
- Not understanding why each medication is needed
- Ignoring side effects without discussion
- Taking over-the-counter drugs without guidance

Red Flag Warnings

Contact your doctor if:

- You develop new symptoms

- You cannot tolerate medications
- You are missing doses frequently
- You feel uncertain about your treatment plan

Key Points

- Medicines reduce the risk of future heart events
- Each medication has a specific role
- Regular use is essential
- Medical guidance ensures safe and effective treatment

Chapter Summary

Long-term medications are a cornerstone of heart disease management. After a heart attack or diagnosis of coronary artery disease, these medicines help prevent clot formation, stabilize plaque, control blood pressure, and protect heart function. While you may feel better after initial treatment, the underlying disease remains. Consistent use of prescribed medications significantly reduces the risk of recurrence and improves long-term outcomes.

Action Plan

- Take all prescribed medications regularly
- Understand the purpose of each medicine

- Do not stop medications without medical advice
- Report side effects promptly
- Keep regular follow-up appointments

Bridge to the Next Chapter

Medicines are essential, but sometimes they are not enough on their own.

In the next chapter, we will discuss procedures such as angioplasty, stents, and bypass surgery, and when they are needed to restore blood flow effectively.

CHAPTER 14: Angioplasty, Stents, and Bypass Surgery – When the Heart Needs More Than Medicines

When Medicines Are Not Enough

For many patients, medicines and lifestyle changes are sufficient to control heart disease.

But in some situations, the narrowing in the coronary arteries becomes significant.

At that point, medicines alone may not provide enough relief or protection.

That is when procedures are considered.

The most common options are:

- Angioplasty
- Stent placement
- Bypass surgery

These may sound complex, but once you understand them, they become much easier to accept.

What Is Angioplasty

Angioplasty is a procedure used to open a narrowed or blocked coronary artery.

A thin tube called a catheter is inserted through a blood vessel, usually from the wrist or groin, and guided to the heart.

At the site of blockage:

- A small balloon is inflated
- The artery is widened
- Blood flow improves

This procedure is commonly used during a heart attack or when significant blockage is found.

What Is a Stent

In most cases, a stent is placed during angioplasty.

A stent is a small mesh tube that:

- Keeps the artery open
- Prevents it from narrowing again
- Helps maintain blood flow

Modern stents are often coated with medication to reduce the risk of future blockage.

STENT VS BYPASS —
TWO WAYS TO RESTORE BLOOD FLOW

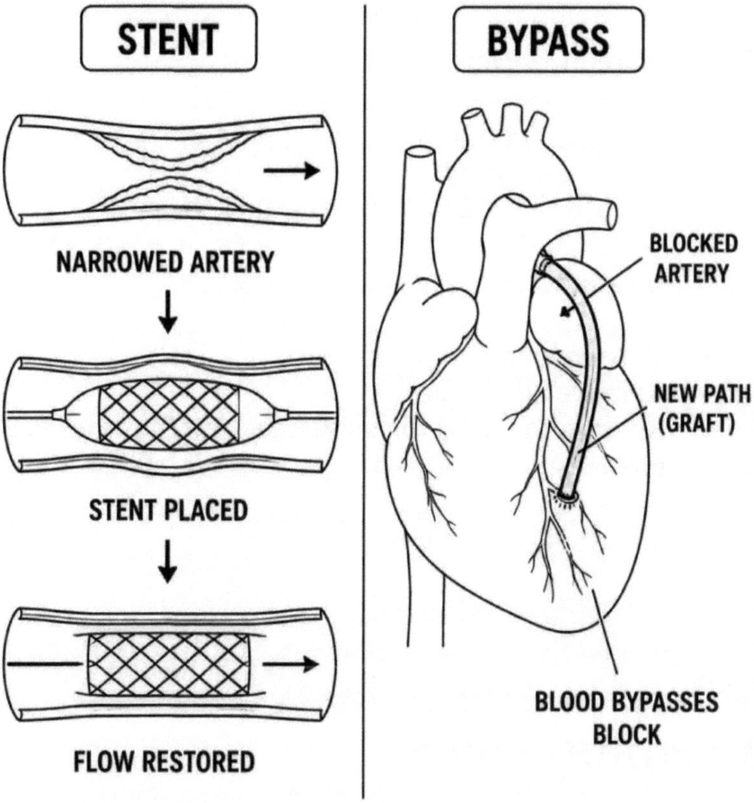

TAKEAWAY:
STENT OPENS THE ARTERY.
BYPASS CREATES A NEW ROUTE.

What These Procedures Can and Cannot Do

It is important to understand both sides.

These procedures can:

- Restore blood flow
- Relieve symptoms
- Reduce risk during a heart attack

But they cannot:

- Cure coronary artery disease
- Remove all plaque
- Replace the need for medicines and lifestyle changes

This distinction is essential.

When Is Angioplasty Recommended

Angioplasty is usually recommended when:

- There is an ongoing heart attack
- Significant blockage is causing symptoms
- Tests show reduced blood flow

The decision depends on:

- Severity of blockage
- Location of narrowing
- Symptoms
- Overall health

What Is Bypass Surgery

Bypass surgery, also called CABG, is a more extensive procedure.

Instead of opening the blocked artery, a new pathway is created for blood flow.

This is done by:

- Taking a healthy blood vessel from another part of the body
- Connecting it to bypass the blocked area

Blood then flows around the blockage.

When Is Bypass Surgery Needed

Bypass surgery is usually recommended when:

- Multiple arteries are severely blocked
- Blockages are complex
- The main coronary artery is involved
- Diabetes is present with widespread disease

In these cases, surgery often provides better long-term results.

Recovery After These Procedures

Recovery depends on the treatment.

After Angioplasty and Stent

- Short hospital stay
- Faster recovery
- Return to normal activities within a few days

After Bypass Surgery

- Longer hospital stay
- Recovery over several weeks
- Gradual return to daily activities

Both require ongoing care and follow-up.

Life After the Procedure — The Real Work Begins

Many patients feel that once a procedure is done, the problem is solved.

That is not correct.

The procedure treats a blockage, but the disease remains.

This means:

- Medicines must continue
- Lifestyle changes are essential
- Follow-up is necessary

Think of the procedure as a repair, not a cure.

A Real-Life Perspective

One patient undergoes angioplasty and feels better, but stops medications and ignores lifestyle changes.

Within months, symptoms return.

Another patient follows all advice:

- Takes medications regularly
- Improves lifestyle
- Attends follow-up

He remains stable and active.

The difference is not the procedure.

The difference is what happens afterward.

Doctor's Pearl

A stent opens an artery, but it does not cure heart disease.

Common Mistakes to Avoid

- Stopping blood-thinning medications after a stent
- Ignoring lifestyle changes
- Missing follow-up visits
- Assuming the problem is permanently fixed

Red Flag Warnings

Seek medical attention if:

- Chest pain returns
- Symptoms worsen
- You feel breathless or unusually tired
- There are concerns about medications

Key Points

- Procedures are used when blockages are significant
- Angioplasty and stents restore blood flow
- Bypass surgery creates a new route for blood flow
- Long-term care remains essential

Chapter Summary

When coronary artery disease leads to significant blockage, procedures such as angioplasty, stenting, and bypass surgery may be required. These treatments improve blood flow, relieve symptoms, and in emergency situations can save lives. However, they do not cure the underlying disease. Long-term success depends on continued medication, lifestyle changes, and regular follow-up.

Action Plan

- Understand why a procedure is recommended
- Follow all post-procedure instructions
- Take medications regularly
- Maintain a heart-healthy lifestyle
- Keep all follow-up appointments

Bridge to the Next Chapter

Even after successful treatment, complications can occur if the disease is not well controlled.

In the next chapter, we will discuss the possible complications of heart disease and how they can affect both the heart and the rest of the body.

CHAPTER 15: Complications of Coronary Artery Disease — What Can Go Wrong and How to Prevent It

Why This Chapter Matters

After treatment, many patients feel relieved.

The immediate danger has passed. The pain is gone. Life begins to feel normal again.

But coronary artery disease is not a one-time problem.

It is a long-term condition.

If not managed properly, it can lead to complications that affect not only the heart, but the entire body.

I am not sharing this to create fear.

I am sharing this so you understand something important:

Most complications can be reduced or prevented with proper care.

Recurrent Heart Attack — The Risk Remains

After one heart attack, the risk of another increases.

This happens because:

- The underlying disease is still present
- Plaque may exist in other arteries
- Risk factors may still be active

Without proper management, the process can repeat.

Each new heart attack may cause additional damage.

Heart Failure — When the Heart Becomes Weak

Heart failure is one of the most common complications.

It occurs when:

- A portion of the heart muscle is damaged
- The heart cannot pump effectively

Symptoms may include:

- Shortness of breath
- Fatigue
- Swelling in the legs
- Reduced exercise capacity

This condition may develop gradually after a heart attack.

Abnormal Heart Rhythms — Electrical Instability

Damage to the heart muscle can affect its electrical system.

This can lead to:

- Irregular heartbeats
- Very fast or very slow rhythms

Symptoms may include:

- Palpitations
- Dizziness
- Fainting

Some rhythm disturbances can be serious.

Sudden Cardiac Arrest — A Critical Emergency

In some cases, abnormal heart rhythms can cause the heart to stop suddenly.

This is called sudden cardiac arrest.

It may occur:

- During a heart attack
- After significant heart damage

Immediate emergency care is required.

Cardiogenic Shock — When the Heart Cannot Support the Body

This is a rare but severe complication.

It occurs when:

- The heart is too weak to pump enough blood
- Vital organs do not receive adequate circulation

This condition requires intensive medical care.

Effects on Other Organs

Heart disease can affect multiple organs.

- Brain → increased risk of stroke
- Kidneys → reduced function
- Lungs → fluid buildup causing breathlessness

The body functions as an interconnected system. When the heart is affected, other organs can also be impacted.

COMPLICATIONS OF CAD

1. HEART ATTACK

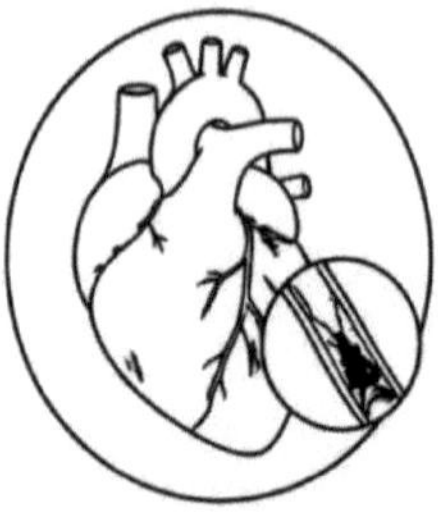

Blocked artery leads to damage of heart muscle.

2. HEART FAILURE

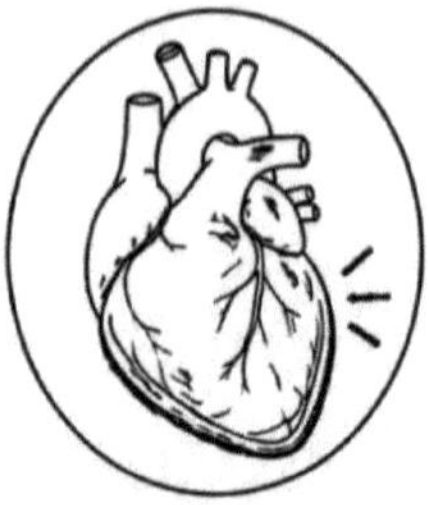

Heart becomes weak and cannot pump blood effectively.

3. ARRHYTHMIA

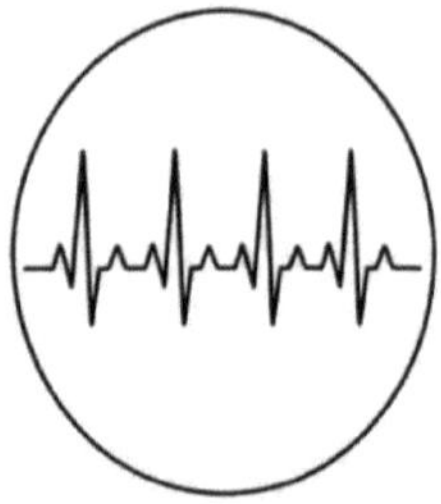

Irregular heart rhythm that can cause dizziness, fainting, or sudden cardiac arrest.

4. SUDDEN CARDIAC DEATH

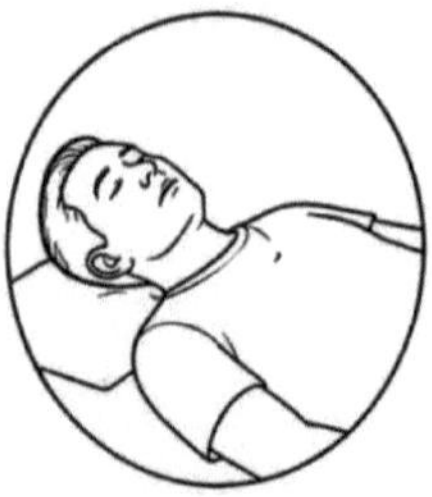

Unexpected death due to severe heart rhythm problems.

5. VALVE PROBLEMS

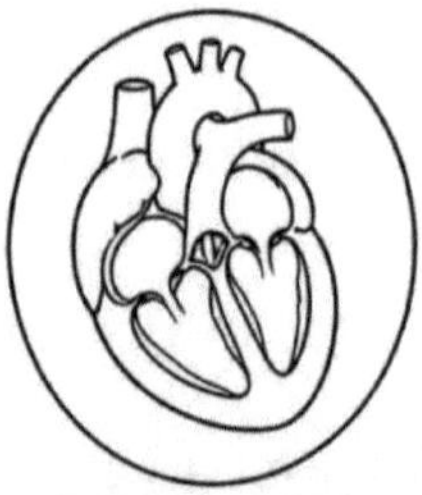

Poor blood flow can affect heart valves and their function.

6. STROKE

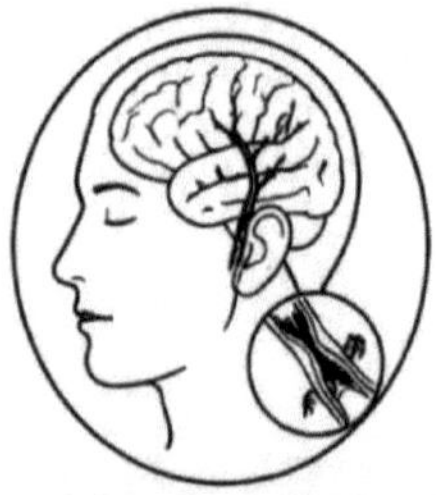

Reduced blood flow or clots can block arteries in the brain.

TAKEAWAY:
Early detection and proper treatment of CAD can prevent these serious complications and save lives.

Emotional and Mental Health Impact

After a heart event, emotional changes are common.

Patients may experience:

- Anxiety
- Fear of recurrence
- Depression

These feelings are real and important.

They can affect:

- Recovery
- Medication adherence
- Quality of life

Addressing emotional health is an essential part of recovery.

Impact on Daily Life

If complications develop, daily life can be affected.

Patients may experience:

- Reduced physical capacity
- Dependence on medications
- Frequent medical visits

This is why prevention is so important.

A Real-Life Perspective

I have seen two very different outcomes.

One patient follows medical advice carefully:

- Takes medications regularly
- Maintains a healthy lifestyle
- Attends follow-up visits

He remains stable and active.

Another patient neglects care:

- Stops medications
- Ignores risk factors

He develops complications.

The difference is not chance.

The difference is consistent care.

Doctor's Pearl

Most complications of heart disease can be prevented or delayed with proper long-term care.

Common Mistakes to Avoid

- Ignoring follow-up care
- Stopping medications
- Returning to unhealthy habits
- Underestimating the seriousness of the condition
- Ignoring early warning signs

Red Flag Warnings

Seek medical attention if you notice:

- Increasing shortness of breath
- Swelling in the legs or abdomen
- Irregular heartbeat
- Sudden dizziness or fainting
- Recurrence of chest discomfort

Key Points

- Coronary artery disease can lead to serious complications
- Heart failure and arrhythmias are common outcomes
- Other organs may also be affected
- Prevention is possible with proper care

Chapter Summary

Coronary artery disease can lead to significant complications if not properly managed. These include recurrent heart attacks, heart failure, abnormal heart rhythms, and effects on other organs. Emotional health may also be affected. However, with proper treatment, lifestyle changes, and regular follow-up, many of these complications can be prevented. Understanding these risks highlights the importance of consistent, long-term care.

Action Plan

- Follow your treatment plan carefully
- Take medications regularly
- Monitor for new or worsening symptoms
- Maintain regular follow-up
- Continue heart-healthy lifestyle habits

Bridge to the Next Chapter

While complications are possible, many patients recover well and return to active lives.

In the next chapter, we will focus on recovery after a heart attack and how to rebuild your strength, confidence, and daily routine step by step.

CHAPTER 16: Recovery After a Heart Attack — A Practical Path Back to Strength and Confidence

The Beginning of a New Phase

When a heart attack is over and you are discharged from the hospital, a new phase begins.

Many patients feel relief.

But along with relief, there is uncertainty.

Questions naturally arise:

- Can I return to a normal life
- Is my heart permanently damaged
- How careful should I be

These are honest concerns.

Let me reassure you clearly.

Most patients can return to a full and active life.

But recovery requires a thoughtful and steady approach.

Recovery Begins Before You Go Home

Your recovery does not begin at home. It begins in the hospital.

During this time, your medical team:

- Stabilizes your condition
- Adjusts medications
- Evaluates heart function
- Educates you about warning signs
- Plans your follow-up care

This is also when your long-term treatment strategy is established.

Do not hesitate to ask questions.

Understanding your plan builds confidence.

The First Few Weeks at Home

The early phase of recovery is important.

You may experience:

- Fatigue
- Reduced stamina
- Mild discomfort
- Emotional ups and downs

This is normal.

Your heart and body are healing.

During this period:

- Rest is important
- Activity should be gradual
- Medications must be taken regularly

Do not rush recovery, but do not remain inactive.

Cardiac Rehabilitation — A Key Part of Recovery

Cardiac rehabilitation is one of the most valuable parts of recovery.

It includes:

- Supervised exercise
- Education about heart health
- Guidance on diet and lifestyle
- Emotional support

Patients who participate often:

- Recover faster
- Feel more confident
- Have fewer complications

If available, this program should be strongly considered.

Returning to Physical Activity

Activity should be resumed gradually.

Start with:

- Short walks
- Light daily activities

Then slowly increase:

- Duration
- Intensity

Avoid:

- Sudden heavy exertion
- Overexertion in the early phase

Consistency is more important than intensity.

Returning to Work and Daily Life

Most patients can return to:

- Work
- Travel
- Social activities

The timing depends on:

- Severity of the heart attack
- Overall health

- Type of work

Your doctor will guide you based on your situation.

Sexual Activity — A Common Concern

Many patients hesitate to discuss this.

In general:

- Sexual activity can be resumed once moderate physical activity can be performed without symptoms

A simple guideline is:

If you can climb two flights of stairs comfortably, you are usually safe.

If you have concerns, discuss them openly with your doctor.

Emotional Recovery — Do Not Ignore It

Emotional changes are common after a heart attack.

You may feel:

- Anxiety
- Fear of recurrence
- Low mood

These feelings are normal.

But they should not be ignored.

Talking with:

- Family
- Friends
- Your doctor

can help significantly.

A Real-Life Perspective

I have seen patients take different approaches.

One becomes overly cautious, avoids activity, and lives in fear. Recovery becomes slow.

Another follows a structured plan, gradually increases activity, and regains confidence.

The second patient recovers better.

The difference is not the severity of the illness.

The difference is the approach to recovery.

RECOVERY AFTER HEART ATTACK

Follow these steps to heal, get stronger, and protect your heart.

1. TAKE MEDICINES AS PRESCRIBED

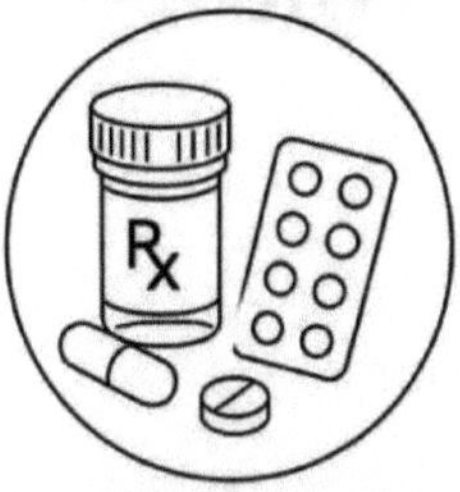

Take all medicines on time. Do not stop without doctor's advice.

2. EAT HEART-HEALTHY FOOD

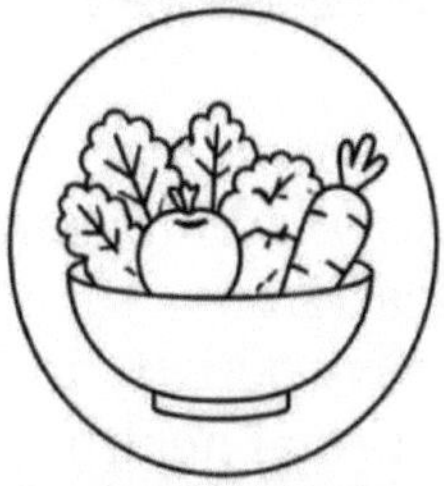

Choose fruits, vegetables, whole grains, lean protein, and low-salt foods.

3. BE PHYSICALLY ACTIVE

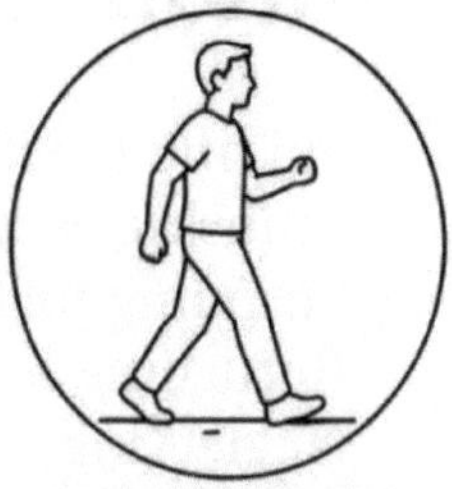

Start with light activity and gradually increase. Aim for 30 minutes most days.

4. STOP SMOKING AND AVOID ALCOHOL

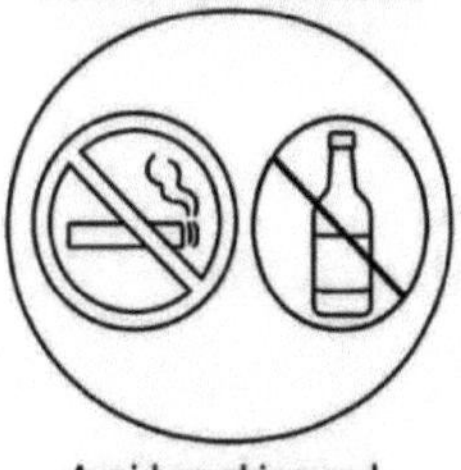

Avoid smoking and limit or avoid alcohol to protect your heart.

5. MANAGE STRESS AND REST WELL

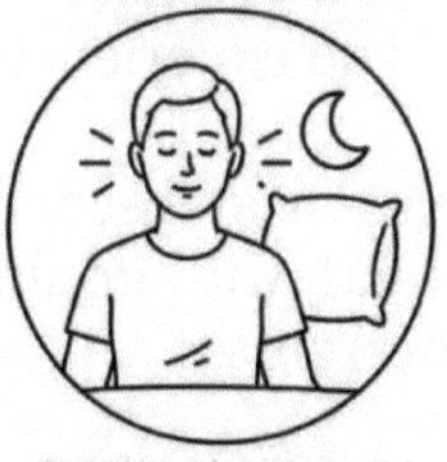

Practice relaxation, get enough sleep, and keep a positive outlook.

6. KEEP REGULAR FOLLOW-UPS

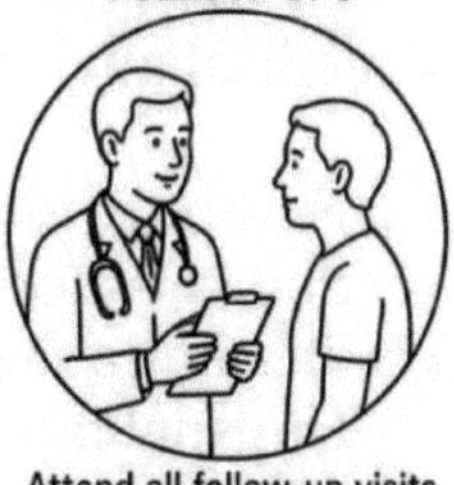

Attend all follow-up visits and tests to monitor your recovery.

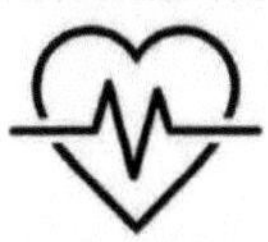

TAKEAWAY

Recovering from a heart attack is a journey. Healthy habits, medicines, and regular care help you live a longer, healthier life.

Doctor's Pearl

Recovery is not about avoiding activity. It is about returning to activity safely and steadily.

Common Mistakes to Avoid

- Staying inactive due to fear
- Ignoring cardiac rehabilitation
- Stopping medications
- Returning to heavy activity too soon
- Neglecting emotional health

Red Flag Warnings

Seek medical advice if you experience:

- New or recurring chest discomfort
- Shortness of breath with minimal activity
- Palpitations or dizziness
- Unusual fatigue

Key Points

- Recovery is gradual and structured

- Cardiac rehabilitation is highly beneficial
- Physical and emotional recovery go together
- Most patients can return to normal life

Chapter Summary

Recovery after a heart attack is a critical phase that determines long-term outcomes. It involves gradual return to activity, adherence to medications, participation in cardiac rehabilitation, and attention to emotional health. With proper guidance and consistent effort, most patients can regain strength, confidence, and quality of life.

Action Plan

- Follow discharge instructions carefully
- Take medications regularly
- Participate in cardiac rehabilitation
- Begin gradual physical activity
- Address emotional concerns
- Keep all follow-up appointments

Bridge to the Next Chapter

Recovery is only the beginning.

In the next chapter, we will focus on daily habits that protect your heart long term, including diet, exercise, sleep, and stress management.

CHAPTER 17: Food, Exercise, Sleep, and Stress — Your Daily Plan to Protect Your Heart

Where Long-Term Health Is Truly Built

After the emergency, the tests, and the treatments, many patients ask a simple question:

"What else can I do to protect my heart?"

My answer is always the same.

What you do every day matters more than what happens occasionally in the hospital.

Your daily habits quietly shape your future.

They can either:

- Protect your heart
  or
- Slowly damage it over time

The encouraging part is this:

You do not need perfection. You need consistency.

Food — The Foundation of Heart Health

Diet is not about strict rules or temporary plans.

It is about a pattern you can follow for life.

A heart-friendly eating pattern includes:

- Fresh vegetables and fruits
- Whole grains
- Nuts and seeds
- Healthy oils such as olive oil
- Lean proteins such as fish, beans, and lentils

Try to limit:

- Processed foods
- Sugary drinks
- Excess salt
- Foods high in saturated and trans fats

Small changes are more effective than drastic ones.

For example:

- Add one extra serving of vegetables daily
- Replace sugary drinks with water
- Reduce portion sizes

Over time, these become natural habits.

Exercise — A Powerful Natural Medicine

Regular physical activity strengthens the heart.

It helps:

- Improve blood circulation
- Lower blood pressure
- Improve blood sugar control
- Reduce stress
- Maintain a healthy weight

A practical goal for most people is:

- About 30 minutes of moderate activity on most days

This can include:

- Walking
- Cycling
- Swimming
- Light jogging

If you are recovering from a heart event, start slowly and build gradually.

Consistency is more important than intensity.

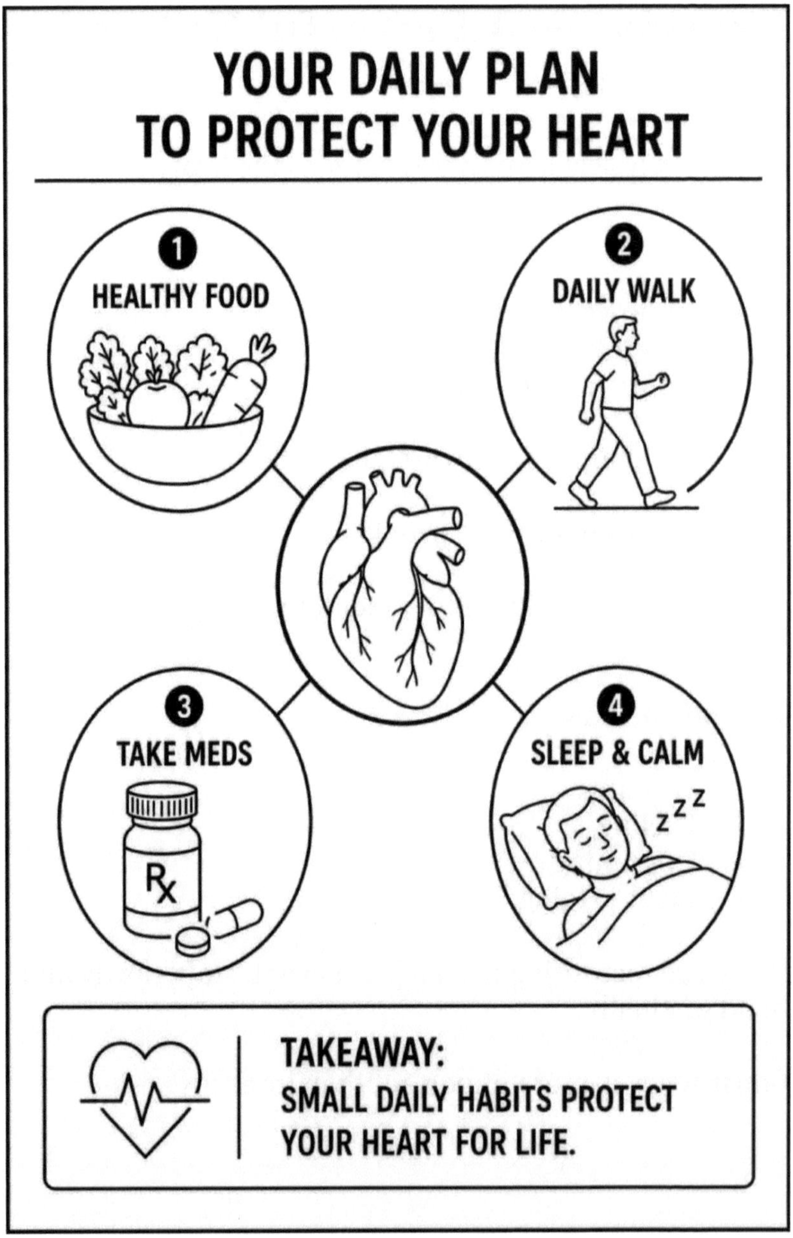

YOUR DAILY PLAN
TO PROTECT YOUR HEART
1
HEALTHY FOOD
2
DAILY WALK
3
TAKE MEDS
Rx
4
SLEEP & CALM
z z z
TAKEAWAY:
SMALL DAILY HABITS PROTECT
YOUR HEART FOR LIFE.

Weight — Focus on Health, Not Just Numbers

Excess weight increases the workload on the heart.

Even modest weight loss can:

- Improve blood pressure
- Improve blood sugar
- Improve cholesterol levels

Avoid extreme diets.

Focus on:

- Sustainable habits
- Regular activity

Healthy weight is about improving function, not appearance.

Sleep — The Overlooked Healer

Sleep plays a major role in heart health.

Poor sleep can:

- Raise blood pressure
- Affect blood sugar
- Increase appetite
- Worsen stress

Most adults need:

- 7 to 8 hours of good-quality sleep

If you:

- Snore loudly
- Feel tired during the day
- Wake up frequently

you may need evaluation for sleep disorders such as sleep apnea.

Stress — The Hidden Contributor

Stress is part of life, but chronic stress can harm the heart.

It can:

- Raise blood pressure
- Affect heart rhythm
- Lead to unhealthy habits

Managing stress does not mean eliminating it.

It means responding to it in a healthier way.

Helpful approaches include:

- Regular physical activity

- Relaxation techniques
- Spending time with loved ones
- Engaging in hobbies

Even small periods of calm can make a difference.

Smoking — The Most Important Change

If you smoke, stopping is the most powerful step you can take.

Smoking:

- Damages blood vessels
- Promotes clot formation
- Reduces oxygen supply

There is no safe level.

The benefits of quitting begin quickly and increase over time.

Alcohol — Keep It Moderate

Excess alcohol can:

- Raise blood pressure
- Affect heart rhythm
- Add unnecessary calories

If you drink, do so in moderation.

If you do not drink, there is no need to start.

A Simple Daily Routine

A heart-healthy day does not have to be complicated.

It may include:

- Balanced meals
- A 30-minute walk
- Adequate hydration
- Time to relax
- Good sleep

These simple steps, repeated daily, create powerful long-term benefits.

A Real-Life Perspective

I have seen patients make small, steady changes.

They walk daily, improve their diet, and manage stress.

Over time, their health improves significantly.

Others rely only on medications without lifestyle changes.

Their progress is limited.

Lifestyle is not optional. It is essential.

Doctor's Pearl

You do not need drastic changes. You need steady, sustainable habits.

Common Mistakes to Avoid

- Starting extreme diets that cannot be maintained
- Exercising too aggressively and then stopping
- Ignoring sleep quality
- Underestimating stress
- Relying only on medications

Red Flag Warnings

Discuss with your doctor if:

- You have symptoms during exercise
- You are unsure how to begin activity
- You have persistent sleep problems
- Stress feels overwhelming

Key Points

- Daily habits shape long-term heart health
- Small consistent changes make a big difference
- Lifestyle and medication work together
- Prevention is an ongoing process

Chapter Summary

Lifestyle is the foundation of heart health. A balanced diet, regular exercise, healthy weight, good sleep, and effective stress management all work together to protect the heart. These are not temporary measures, but long-term habits. When practiced consistently, they significantly reduce the risk of future heart problems and improve overall well-being.

Action Plan

- Follow a balanced, heart-healthy diet
- Exercise regularly
- Maintain a healthy weight
- Improve sleep quality
- Manage stress effectively
- Stop smoking completely

Bridge to the Next Chapter

You now understand how daily habits protect your heart.

In the next chapter, we will focus on one of the most important goals:

How to prevent the next heart attack and maintain long-term heart health with confidence.

CHAPTER 18: Preventing the Next Heart Attack — A Practical, Lifelong Protection Plan

The Question That Matters Most

After recovery, one question stays with almost every patient:

"Will this happen again?"

This is a very real concern.

Let me answer it clearly.

A second heart attack is not inevitable.

With the right plan and consistent effort, your risk can be reduced significantly.

This chapter is about taking control of that risk.

What Is Secondary Prevention

In simple terms, secondary prevention means:

Protecting your heart after a heart problem has already occurred.

It includes:

- Medications
- Lifestyle changes
- Monitoring
- Regular follow-up

This is not a temporary phase.

It is a lifelong strategy.

Why Risk Still Exists

Even after treatment:

- The underlying disease is still present
- Plaque may remain in other arteries
- Risk factors may still be active

But this is not a reason for fear.

It is a reason for action.

Because when you control these factors, you change the course of the disease.

Know Your Numbers — Your Personal Dashboard

Monitoring your health helps you stay in control.

Important numbers include:

- Blood pressure
- LDL cholesterol
- Blood sugar levels
- Body weight and waist size

These numbers guide treatment decisions.

Regular monitoring helps prevent surprises.

Medications — Your Daily Protection

Your medications are not temporary.

They:

- Prevent clot formation
- Stabilize plaque
- Reduce strain on the heart

Stopping medications increases risk.

Even when you feel well, they continue to protect you.

Lifestyle — The Foundation of Prevention

Medications alone are not enough.

Long-term protection depends on:

- Healthy eating
- Regular physical activity
- Weight control
- Good sleep
- Stress management

These are not optional.

They are essential parts of treatment.

Regular Follow-Up — Staying Ahead

Your condition can change over time.

Regular follow-up helps:

- Adjust medications
- Monitor risk factors
- Detect problems early

Think of follow-up visits as preventive care.

Recognizing Early Warning Signs

Remain alert to changes.

Watch for:

- New chest discomfort
- Shortness of breath
- Unusual fatigue

Early recognition allows early action.

Do not ignore subtle symptoms.

Building Habits That Last

Prevention is not about perfection.

It is about consistency.

Simple daily actions matter:

- Taking medications
- Staying active
- Eating wisely
- Monitoring health

Over time, these habits create strong protection.

The Role of Support

Family and support systems are important.

They can help you:

- Stay motivated
- Maintain healthy habits
- Recognize warning signs

You do not have to manage this alone.

A Real-Life Perspective

I have seen patients take two different paths.

One follows advice consistently and remains stable for years.

Another becomes relaxed after recovery, stops medications, and ignores lifestyle changes.

The risk returns.

The difference is not luck.

The difference is commitment.

Doctor's Pearl

Prevention begins the moment your first heart problem is treated.

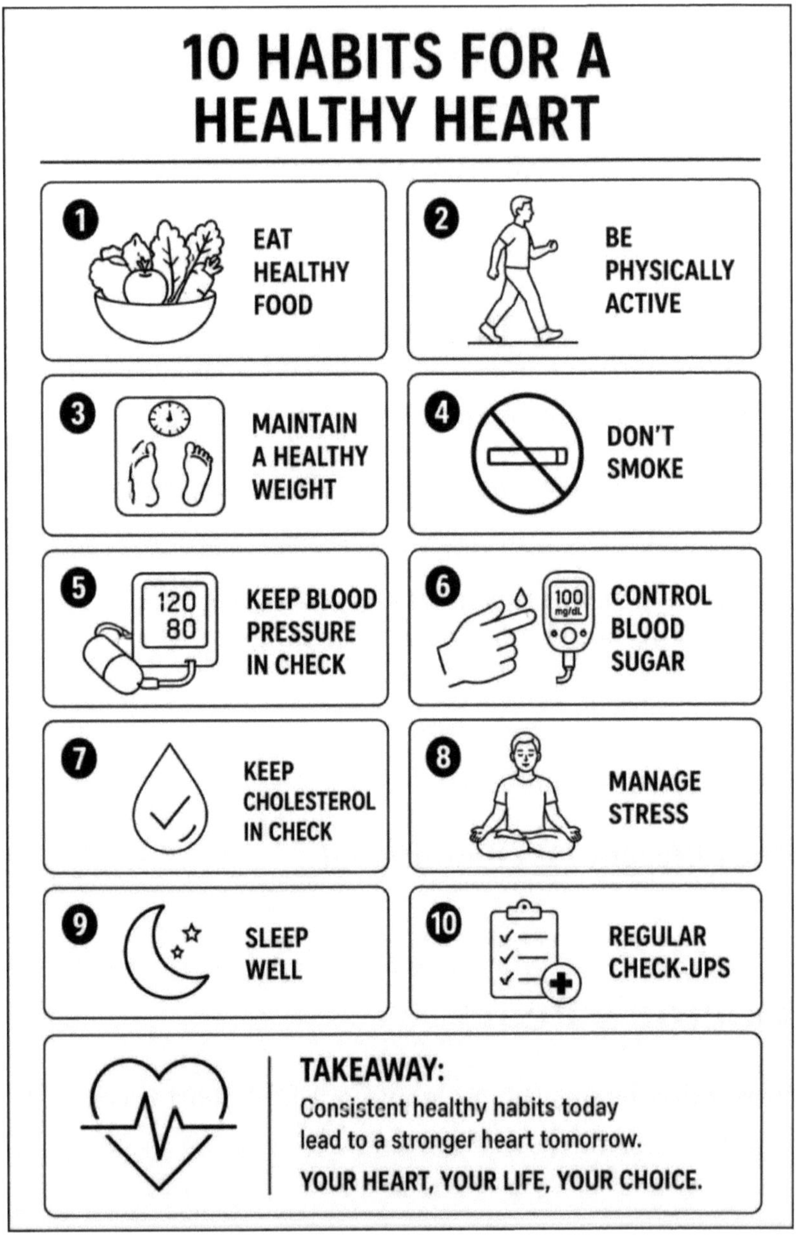
10 HABITS FOR A HEALTHY HEART
1
EAT HEALTHY FOOD
2
BE PHYSICALLY ACTIVE
3
MAINTAIN A HEALTHY WEIGHT
4
DON'T SMOKE
5
120
80
KEEP BLOOD PRESSURE IN CHECK
6
100
mg/dL
CONTROL BLOOD SUGAR
7
KEEP CHOLESTEROL IN CHECK
8
MANAGE STRESS
9
SLEEP WELL
10
REGULAR CHECK-UPS
TAKEAWAY:
Consistent healthy habits today lead to a stronger heart tomorrow.
YOUR HEART, YOUR LIFE, YOUR CHOICE.

Common Mistakes to Avoid

- Becoming relaxed after recovery
- Stopping medications
- Ignoring follow-up
- Returning to unhealthy habits
- Not monitoring health

Red Flag Warnings

Seek medical advice if:

- Symptoms return or worsen
- You are unsure about medications
- Risk factors are not controlled
- You feel uncertain about your plan

Key Points

- Secondary prevention reduces recurrence risk
- Monitoring health is essential
- Medications and lifestyle work together
- Consistency is the key to success

Chapter Summary

Preventing a second heart attack is a central goal after recovery. Although the underlying disease may remain, it can be effectively controlled through medications, lifestyle changes, and regular follow-up. Monitoring health parameters and recognizing early warning signs further strengthen protection. With consistent effort, you can significantly reduce your risk and maintain a healthy and active life.

Action Plan

- Monitor your health regularly
- Take medications as prescribed
- Maintain a heart-healthy lifestyle
- Attend regular follow-up visits
- Act early if symptoms change

Bridge to the Next Chapter

Medicine continues to evolve and offer new tools for better care.

In the next chapter, we will explore recent advances in heart care and what they mean for you.

CHAPTER 19: Newer Tests, Newer Treatments, and the Future of Heart Care — What You Should Know

A Quiet Revolution in Heart Care

If I look back over the years, the change in heart care has been remarkable.

Diagnoses are faster.
Treatments are safer.
Recovery is smoother.

Many patients who once required major surgery can now be treated through a small tube placed in the wrist.

But let me say something clearly at the beginning:

New technology helps, but it does not replace the basics.

Understanding what is new, and how it fits into your care, will help you make better decisions.

Advanced Imaging — Seeing the Problem More Clearly

Modern imaging has improved the way we diagnose heart disease.

Coronary CT Angiography

This test provides detailed images of the coronary arteries without invasive procedures.

It helps:

- Detect narrowing early
- Identify plaque
- Guide treatment decisions

Improved Echocardiography

Today's echocardiograms provide clearer and more detailed information.

They help assess:

- Heart function
- Valve problems
- Subtle abnormalities

Better Imaging Overall

Modern imaging allows doctors to:

- Detect disease earlier
- Avoid unnecessary invasive tests

- Make more accurate decisions

Calcium Scoring — Detecting Risk Early

Calcium scoring is a simple scan that measures calcium deposits in the coronary arteries.

It helps:

- Identify early plaque buildup
- Estimate long-term risk
- Guide preventive strategies

This test is most useful in people without symptoms but with risk factors.

Newer Cholesterol-Lowering Treatments

Statins remain the foundation.

But newer options are now available:

- Injectable medications that significantly lower LDL
- Additional drugs for patients who cannot tolerate statins
- Combination therapies for high-risk individuals

These provide more flexibility and improved control.

Improved Blood-Thinning Strategies

Newer medications allow better balance between:

- Preventing clots
- Reducing bleeding risk

Treatment can now be tailored more precisely to each patient.

Personalized Treatment — Care That Fits You

One of the most important advances is individualized care.

Instead of a one-size-fits-all approach:

- Treatment is tailored to your risk
- Decisions are based on detailed data
- Care is adjusted over time

This improves outcomes and safety.

Wearable Technology — Monitoring Beyond the Clinic

Technology now allows patients to track their health at home.

Devices such as:

- Smart watches
- Home blood pressure monitors
- Fitness trackers

can help:

- Monitor heart rate
- Track activity
- Detect rhythm changes

These tools increase awareness and engagement.

But they should support, not replace, medical care.

Minimally Invasive Procedures — Faster Recovery

Procedures have become less invasive.

Advances include:

- Better stents
- Improved catheter techniques

- Shorter recovery times

Patients often:

- Experience less discomfort
- Return to normal activity sooner

What Is Still Evolving

Some areas are still developing:

- Advanced plaque imaging
- Genetic risk assessment
- Anti-inflammatory treatments

These may play a larger role in the future.

What Has Not Changed

Despite all these advances, some principles remain constant:

- Healthy lifestyle
- Risk factor control
- Medication adherence

These continue to form the foundation of heart health.

A Real-Life Perspective

Some patients rely heavily on technology but ignore lifestyle changes.

Others use technology as a support while maintaining healthy habits.

The second approach leads to better long-term outcomes.

Doctor's Pearl

Technology supports your health, but daily habits determine your future.

Common Mistakes to Avoid

- Relying only on new tests
- Ignoring lifestyle changes
- Misinterpreting device data
- Expecting new treatments to replace basic care

Red Flag Warnings

Discuss with your doctor if:

- Device readings are abnormal

- You are considering new treatments
- You are unsure about test results

Key Points

- Advances have improved diagnosis and treatment
- New medications offer additional options
- Technology helps monitor health
- Basic principles remain essential

Chapter Summary

Modern cardiology has made significant progress in diagnosing and treating heart disease. Advanced imaging, newer medications, personalized care, and wearable technology have improved patient outcomes and engagement. However, these advances complement, rather than replace, the fundamentals of heart health. A balanced approach that combines modern medicine with healthy lifestyle habits provides the best long-term results.

Action Plan

- Stay informed about your health
- Use technology wisely
- Follow evidence-based treatment
- Maintain healthy habits

- Discuss new options with your doctor

Bridge to the Final Chapter

You have now understood the journey from symptoms to diagnosis, treatment, and prevention.

In the final chapter, we will bring everything together, address common myths, and leave you with a clear and confident path forward.

CHAPTER 20: Myths, FAQs, and Final Advice — Taking Charge of Your Heart Health

Clearing Confusion and Building Confidence

By now, you have walked through the full journey.

You understand:

- What chest pain can mean
- When it is an emergency
- How heart disease develops
- How it is diagnosed and treated
- How to recover and prevent future problems

But in real life, patients are surrounded by mixed messages.

Friends offer advice.
The internet adds confusion.
Old beliefs continue to circulate.

This final chapter is meant to bring clarity.

Let us separate myth from fact and focus on what truly protects your heart.

Common Myths — And the Truth

"If my ECG is normal, my heart is fine"

This is not always true.

An ECG shows the heart's electrical activity at a moment in time. Many patients with heart disease may have a normal ECG, especially early on.

"If the pain improves with antacids, it must be acidity"

Not necessarily.

Heart-related discomfort can sometimes improve temporarily.

Never rely on this as proof that the heart is not involved.

"Heart attacks are always severe and dramatic"

This is a dangerous misconception.

Many heart attacks are mild, silent, or present with unusual symptoms such as fatigue or breathlessness.

“Once I have a stent, I am cured”

A stent treats a blockage.

It does not cure the disease.

Medications and lifestyle changes remain essential.

“I feel fine, so I do not need follow-up”

Heart disease can progress silently.

Regular follow-up helps detect problems early.

“Medicines are only needed for a short time”

Most heart medications are long-term.

They protect you even when you feel well.

Frequently Asked Questions

Can I live a normal life after a heart attack

Yes.

With proper treatment, rehabilitation, and lifestyle changes, most patients return to active and fulfilling lives.

Is exercise safe

Yes, and it is encouraged.

It should be started gradually and guided by your doctor.

Can I travel

In most cases, yes.

Once your condition is stable, travel is generally safe. Discuss long trips with your doctor.

Can I return to work

Most patients can.

The timing depends on your recovery and the nature of your work.

Is every chest pain dangerous

No.

But any new, unusual, or persistent chest discomfort should be evaluated.

How long will I need medications

Many medications are long-term.

Your doctor will guide you based on your condition.

Bringing It All Together

Let us step back and look at the big picture.

Heart disease is common.

But it is also manageable.

You now understand:

- The warning signs
- The risk factors
- The treatment options
- The importance of prevention

This knowledge gives you control.

It replaces fear with understanding.

A Simple Daily Checklist

A practical daily routine can make a real difference:

- Take medications regularly
- Stay physically active
- Eat balanced meals
- Get adequate sleep
- Manage stress
- Stay aware of symptoms

These simple steps, practiced consistently, create lasting benefits.

Your Role in Your Own Care

Your doctor provides guidance.

Medicines provide protection.

Procedures provide support.

But your daily choices determine your long-term outcome.

Think of your care as a partnership.

- Medicine provides the tools
- You provide the consistency

A Real-Life Perspective

Over the years, I have seen two types of patients.

Some take their condition seriously.

They follow advice, make steady changes, and stay engaged.

They do well.

Others ignore early signs, stop medications, and delay follow-up.

Their outcomes are very different.

The difference is not knowledge alone.

The difference is action.

Doctor's Pearl

Your daily habits matter more than occasional medical visits.

Common Mistakes to Avoid

- Ignoring warning signs
- Believing common myths
- Stopping medications without advice

- Neglecting lifestyle changes
- Skipping follow-up

Red Flag Warnings

Seek medical attention if:

- Chest discomfort returns or changes
- You develop breathlessness or unusual fatigue
- You feel uncertain about your symptoms

Key Points

- Many myths about heart disease are misleading
- Understanding facts improves decision-making
- Consistent care prevents complications
- You can take control of your heart health

Chapter Summary

Heart disease can feel overwhelming, but it is manageable with the right approach. Misunderstandings and myths often lead to delay and poor outcomes. By understanding the facts, recognizing warning signs, and following a consistent plan of treatment and lifestyle changes, you can significantly reduce your risk and improve your quality of life. Knowledge combined with action is the key to long-term heart health.

Final Action Plan

- Stay informed and aware
- Take medications as prescribed
- Maintain healthy daily habits
- Monitor your symptoms
- Keep regular follow-up appointments
- Act early when warning signs appear

Closing Message

Chest pain can be frightening.

Heart disease can feel overwhelming.

But you are not powerless.

With the right knowledge, timely action, and consistent care, you can protect your heart and live a full and active life.

This is not just about avoiding disease.

It is about building a healthier future, one day at a time.

End of Book

APPENDIX A: A Simple Daily Heart Health Routine

Turning Knowledge Into Daily Action

Many patients understand what to do, but struggle with how to apply it in daily life.

This simple routine is designed to make heart care practical, realistic, and sustainable.

You do not need perfection.
You need consistency.

Morning — Setting the Tone for the Day

- Wake up at a regular time
- Take your prescribed medications
- Check blood pressure if advised
- Eat a balanced breakfast such as oatmeal, fruit, or eggs with whole grain toast
- Take a short walk or do gentle stretching

A steady start creates a steady day.

Midday — Staying Balanced

- Eat a balanced lunch with vegetables, lean protein, and whole grains
- Stay well hydrated
- Avoid heavy and oily meals
- Take a short walk after meals if possible

Small movement after meals improves overall health.

Evening — Slowing Down

- Eat a lighter dinner, preferably earlier in the evening
- Avoid overeating
- Take a relaxed walk after dinner
- Spend time with family or engage in calming activities

This is the time to reduce both physical and mental stress.

Night — Supporting Recovery

- Avoid screens before bedtime
- Keep your sleep environment calm and comfortable
- Aim for 7 to 8 hours of good-quality sleep

Sleep is when your body repairs itself.

Weekly Goals

- At least 150 minutes of moderate activity per week
- Monitor your weight
- Review your eating habits
- Plan meals for the coming week

Doctor's Pearl

A simple routine followed daily is more powerful than occasional effort.

APPENDIX B: What To Do During Chest Pain — A Clear Emergency Plan

Why This Matters

In a moment of chest discomfort, confusion and delay are common.

A clear plan can save time and save lives.

Step 1: Recognize the Symptoms

Be alert for:

- Chest pressure, tightness, or heaviness
- Pain spreading to the arm, jaw, neck, back, or upper abdomen
- Shortness of breath
- Sweating, nausea, or dizziness

Step 2: Stop and Rest

- Stop all activity immediately
- Sit or lie down

- Stay as calm as possible

Step 3: Call 911 Without Delay

- Do not wait to see if symptoms improve
- Do not attempt to drive yourself
- Emergency services provide early treatment

Step 4: Take Aspirin if Previously Advised

- Chew one aspirin if your doctor has recommended it
- Do not take if allergic or contraindicated

Step 5: Wait Safely for Help

- Stay with someone if possible
- Keep communication open
- Avoid exertion

What Not To Do

- Do not ignore symptoms
- Do not try home remedies first

- Do not delay calling for help

Doctor's Pearl

When in doubt, treat chest pain as a heart emergency.

APPENDIX C: Understanding Your Key Health Numbers

Why These Numbers Matter

These numbers guide your treatment and prevention.

They help you and your doctor make informed decisions.

Blood Pressure

- Ideal: around 120/80 mmHg
- Elevated: 130/80 mmHg or higher

Regular monitoring is essential.

Cholesterol

- LDL (bad cholesterol): lower is better, often less than 70 mg/dL in high-risk patients
- HDL (good cholesterol): higher is better
- Triglycerides: ideally less than 150 mg/dL

Blood Sugar

- Fasting glucose: less than 100 mg/dL (normal range)
- HbA1c: less than 5.7 percent in non-diabetics, individualized in others

---

Body Weight

- Maintain a healthy weight
- Pay attention to waist size

Doctor's Pearl

Knowing your numbers is the first step toward controlling them.

APPENDIX D: A Practical 30-Day Heart Health Reset Plan

A Short Plan With Long-Term Impact

This 30-day plan helps you build habits that can last for years.

Focus on steady progress, not perfection.

Week 1 — Awareness

- Track your food intake
- Begin 10 to 15 minutes of walking daily
- Check blood pressure if advised
- Reduce sugary drinks

Week 2 — Building Momentum

- Increase walking to 20 to 25 minutes
- Add more fruits and vegetables
- Reduce salt intake
- Improve sleep habits

Week 3 — Strengthening Habits

- Aim for 30 minutes of daily activity
- Reduce processed foods
- Begin simple stress management techniques
- Monitor your weight

Week 4 — Making It Routine

- Maintain a consistent daily schedule
- Review your progress
- Set long-term goals
- Reinforce medication adherence

The Real Goal

This is not just a 30-day plan.

It is the beginning of a lifelong routine.

Doctor's Pearl

Short-term discipline creates long-term freedom from disease.

Thank You and Please Review the Book

Thank you for taking the time to read this book. I sincerely hope it has helped you understand your health a little more clearly and has given you practical, everyday steps you can follow with confidence. If you found this book helpful, **I would truly appreciate it if you could leave a brief and honest review.** Even a few lines sharing your experience can make a meaningful difference. Your feedback helps other readers find reliable, trustworthy health information and supports them in making better decisions for themselves and their families.

Warm regards,

Dr Prabhat Das

Continue your Healthcare Journey with these Books

Good health is a journey, not a single step. It is not achieved in one day or with one book. That is why I created the "Better Health with Dr Das Series", with each book addressing a different common condition. If you would like easy, practical guidance on other everyday health concerns, you may wish to explore the rest of books in this series.

Books in this series:

- Better Health starts Here: A Doctor's Guide to Staying Healthy After 40
- A Doctor's Easy Guide to Understanding & Managing OBESITY
- Doctor, What DIET Is Best for Me?
- Doctor, Why Can't I Lose Weight? A Doctor's Guide to Safe & Sustainable Weight Loss)
- A Doctor's Easy Guide to GLP-1 for Obesity
- A Doctor's Easy Guide to Understanding & Managing HIGH BLOOD PRESSURE
- A Doctor's Guide to Living Well With DIABETES
- A Doctor's Guide to Understanding & Managing THYROID DISEASES
- A Doctor's Guide to Understanding & Managing HIGH CHOLESTEROL
- A Doctor's Practical Guide to HEART HEALTH After 40: How to Protect Your Heart & Live Longer
- A Doctor's Guide to Healing & Reversing FATTY LIVER DISEASE: Simple, Natural & Science-Based Steps to Reduce Liver Fat and Prevent Complications

- Control Your ACID REFLUX, HEARTBURN & GERD: A Doctor's Practical Guide that Works
- Live Comfortably with IRRITABLE BOWEL SYNDROME: A Doctor's Practical Guide to Understanding & Managing IBS
- A Doctor's Practical Guide to Understanding & Managing GALLBLADDER STONES & OTHER PROBLEMS
- Take Control of COPD: A Doctor's Practical Guide to Better Breathing
- Living Better with ASTHMA: A Doctor's Practical Guide to Asthma Control
- SLEEP APNEA, INSOMNIA & OTHER SLEEP DISORDERS: A Doctor's Practical Guide to Better Sleep & Better Health
- Protect Your KIDNEYS: A Doctor's Practical Guide to Kidney Health & Prevention
- PROSTATE HEALTH: A Doctor's Practical Guide to Early Detection & Care
- ARTHRITIS: A Doctor's Practical Guide to Pain Control & Mobility
- STROKE: A Doctor's Practical Guide to Prevention & Early detection
- CHEST PAIN & HEART ATTACK: A Doctor's Guide to Recognizing Warning Signs, Acting Early & Protecting Your Life
- CANCER: A Doctor's Practical Guide to Prevention & Early detection
- BACK PAIN A Doctor's Practical Guide to Fixing Step by Step
- COMMON SKIN & HAIR PROBLEMS: A Doctor's Practical Guide to Skin & Hair Care
- DEMENTIA & MEMORY LOSS: A Doctor's Practical Guide to Prevention & Management

- Doctor, Why Am I TIRED All the Time? Fixing Fatigue & Getting Your Energy Back

Printed by Libri Plureos GmbH in Hamburg,
Germany